THE

PLANT
PARADOX
COOKBOOK

To charity: water—

for your tireless efforts to bring clean water to millions of people who need it.
Because you can go months without food, but only seven days without water!

www.charitywater.org

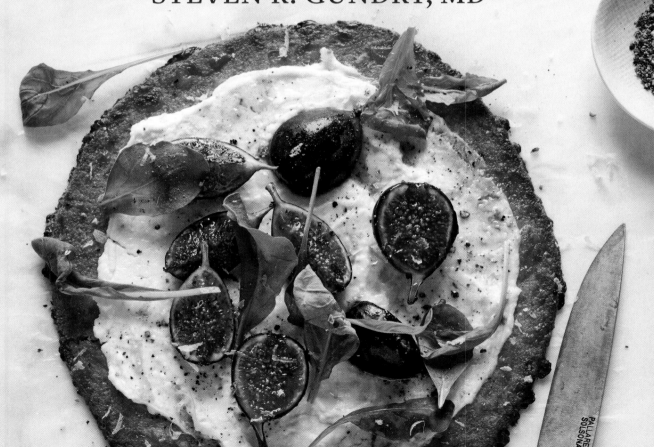

THE

PLANT
PARADOX
COOKBOOK

100 Delicious Recipes to Help You Lose Weight,
Heal Your Gut, and Live Lectin-Free

STEVEN R. GUNDRY, MD

HARPER WAVE

An Imprint of HarperCollins*Publishers*

HarperCollins books may be purchased for educational, business, or sales promotional use. For information, please email the Special Markets Department at SPsales@harpercollins.com.

FIRST EDITION

Photographs © 2018 Dana Gallagher
Produced by Stonesong Press, LLC
Designed by Alison Lew, Vertigo Design
Additional typesetting by Brad Walrod, Kenoza Type, Inc.

Library of Congress Cataloging-in-Publication Data has been applied for.

ISBN 978-0-06-284337-1

19 20 21 22   LSC   20 19 18 17 16 15 14 13 12 11

CONTENTS

Introduction

This cookbook has been a long time in the making. Soon after I began giving my patients a now-infamous list of "just say no" and "yes, please" foods and sent them on their way with about ten recipes, I recognized the need for a more comprehensive resource that could help them maintain their new way of eating. And so for years, I've been collecting recipes from friends and patients and developing my own repertoire. It's taken a lot of trial and error, tasting and testing, and plenty of dirty dishes, but I've finally been able to compile the collection of tasty, healthy, and diverse recipes that my patients—and you readers—deserve.

But let me back up a bit. If you're just coming to this book without having read *The Plant Paradox*, you may be thinking: what is this list you're talking about, and why do I need it? For the past seventeen years, I've been treating patients with a combination of nutritional therapy and conventional medicine. People generally come to see me when they're struggling with a chronic disease and just can't seem to get better. They arrive at one of my clinics—in Palm Springs or Santa Barbara—on a personal journey to regain their health or their loved one's health, or to take their "good enough" health to robust, vibrant health.

As my patients and regular readers know, I saw and continue to see dramatic reversals of diseases I once thought impossible to manage; changes that we can track with sophisticated blood work and that my patients can feel and see. Many of these changes are directly linked to nutritional alterations we've made to their diets. And so I wrote *The Plant Paradox* to explain the philosophy behind the list: the idea that proteins called lectins found in many common "health foods"—including fruits, vegetables, grains, and beans—can damage the gut, cause inflammation, and contribute to disease. Removing major lectin-containing foods from the diet, combined with minimizing exposure to environmental toxins, are the practices at the core of the Plant Paradox program.

The Plant Paradox Cookbook is written first and foremost for all of you who have applied my "rules" and regained your health, but keep finding yourselves asking that immortal question: "What the heck can I eat?" I know that you live in the real world of two-job families, commutes, after-school practices, and socializing, and that relatively few of you reside as I do in Southern California, where beautiful, fresh produce is available year-round. And I know that thinking about going lectin-free can seem impossible, or at least impractical, when you already have too many things to manage on your to-do list. That's why I've written a cookbook with simple recipes anyone can master and accessible ingredients (and substitutions for less-accessible ingredients) you can source easily. I've also incorporated your feedback and suggestions for the types of dishes you most wanted to see. No eating plan that encourages deprivation or sacrifice has ever worked, and for good reason: eating is pleasurable! I of all people understand and appreciate that point—I love a good meal and am not immune to the temptation of my old favorites. That's why you'll find Plant Paradox–approved versions of all of your most-loved foods in these pages, from bagels and pancakes to pizza and pad Thai, spaghetti and meatballs to brownies and ice cream. I know it's hard to believe, but you can reap the benefits of the program while indulging in all of these seemingly forbidden dishes.

That brings me to the second reason for *The Plant Paradox Cookbook*: the Plant Paradox program works! It's just that simple. I've documented it in thousands of patients in my clinics and I've reported my results at major medical conferences, but the real joy I get is when I receive an email or a letter, or read a review online, saying that this program has positively impacted someone's life. Whether it's finally losing weight after many failed attempts; lowering blood pressure and cholesterol markers; improving heart health; reducing or going off of immune-suppressive drugs or thyroid medications; resolving MS or lupus (and the attendant painful symptoms); or slowing or reversing the progression of cancer or

dementia, you've shared so many incredible successes with me that I am truly humbled. Your stories are why I get up and go to work each morning, and why I write books like this one: to make available to everyone the healing powers of the Plant Paradox program.

And lastly, this book is written for you "holdouts" who may have heard about this crazy Plant Paradox thing, but are reluctant to give up your beloved grains and favorite foods. This cookbook was written maybe most of all for you, to make it easier for you to find out what all the fuss is really about and to give this lifestyle a try in the easiest possible way: by making delicious meals.

So, even if you haven't read *The Plant Paradox*, you can jump right in with this book and join the lectin-free (or at least lectin-light) club. Over the next few chapters I'll offer a brief overview of the Plant Paradox plan so that all of us—old hands or newbies alike—will be up to speed and ready to dive into the kitchen!

In case flipping through these pages and catching a glance of the gorgeous photos hasn't persuaded you, let me assure you: I've got incredible dishes from James Beard Award–winning chefs, contributions from my recipe contest at GundryMD.com, and a bunch of out-of-this-world recipes from patients and followers that I know you will love. And they were all made with you, your health, your busy life, and your taste buds in mind. I can't wait for you to try them. Welcome to *The Plant Paradox Cookbook*!

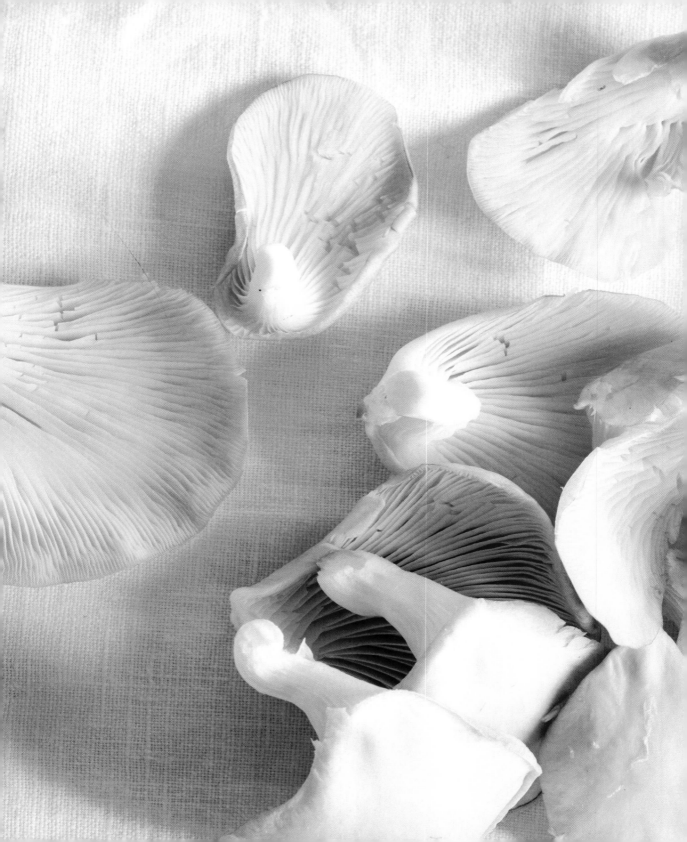

part one

What Is the Plant Paradox?

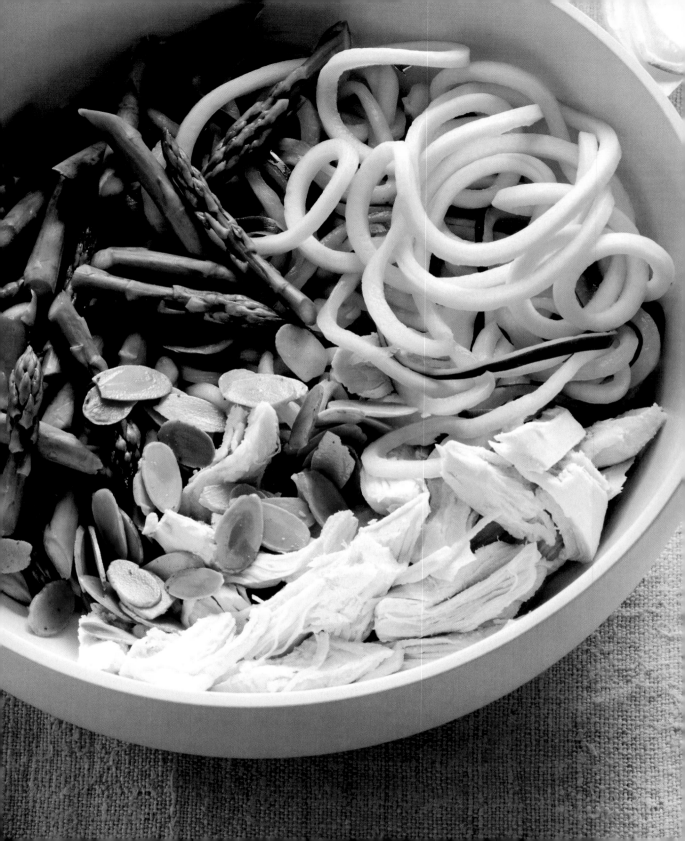

chapter one

Lectins and Your Health

As a clinician, researcher, and former professor, I love to break down complicated science and make it simple and (pardon the pun) digestible.

And one of the simplest principles of healthy eating is this: plants are the cornerstone of a healthy diet. Think of Michael Pollan's elegant summation: "Eat food. Mostly plants. Not too much."

Though I love a straightforward rule, there's another elemental truth that we have to consider: not all plants are good for us.

In fact, certain plants can be harmful to your health, particularly those that contain a type of protein called a lectin, which is designed to cause harm to any creature that consumes the plant. And that's the paradox: plants are both friend *and* enemy, source of health *and*, in certain instances, triggers of disease.

Some plants are more dangerous than others, including many of the plants that have long been considered to be some of the healthiest foods you could eat. Fruit, for example. And vegetables with seeds that are technically fruits (such as cucumbers, tomatoes, squashes, zucchini, and eggplant). Wheat. Corn. Beans and other legumes.

I know what you might be thinking—how could it possibly be true that the fresh, colorful foods in the produce section could actually be *un*healthy? Or that the beans, whole wheat bread, and brown rice we've hailed as health foods for decades could actually cause us harm? Well, to really understand it, we have to do a little time travel. (I bet you didn't expect to read that sentence in a cookbook!)

I want you to imagine that it is 450 million years ago. The only living things on Earth are plants. With no predators, they rule the land, using their incredible chemical ability to transform sunlight into matter to proliferate. Then, about 90 million years later, insects showed up. Suddenly, plants had to develop defensive mechanisms to protect themselves and their babies (aka their seeds) from being eaten, because plants don't want to be killed and consumed any more than you do, and they don't want their babies to be eaten either. Like all life forms, they are programmed to grow and reproduce, and being eaten puts the kibosh on all these biological imperatives.

Since the arrival of insects, plants have been developing and refining sophisticated ways to prevent other creatures—including humans, who first began to evolve only about two to four million years ago—from eating them.

That's 340 million years of evolution that plants have on us; 340 million years of developing defense mechanisms.

You may think that plants are pretty helpless, but they actually possess an impressive arsenal of tactics to protect themselves from predators. For example, while they may not be able to run, they can hide by adapting their color to blend in with their surroundings. And while most plants can't launch an offensive attack, they can defend themselves by causing injury to any creature that eats them. This includes short-term strategies like poisoning, paralyzing, or entrapping their predators. It also includes the long-term strategy of making them very, very sick.

Lectins are a long-term defense strategy. (Gluten is a lectin, you may be surprised to learn, but it's certainly not the only one, nor even the most dangerous. It's just the media darling—the Kim Kardashian—of lectins.) As I mentioned, lectins are proteins—most are large, sticky proteins that are drawn to sugar molecules. When you eat a plant that is high in lectins, one of the negative outcomes is that these proteins start marauding throughout your digestive tract, looking for sugar molecules to which they can hitch their wagon. Your intestinal lining is only about one cell thick. While it is delicate, it is elegantly designed to keep some food particles inside the gut (so they can ultimately be excreted as waste) and to allow the small particles of vitamins, minerals, and other nutrients your body needs to pass through the wall and into the bloodstream. It does this through a series of tight junctions that function as gatekeepers between the cells in the lining of your gut.

The way these tight junctions function is similar to a game of Red Rover—when a line of little kids locks arms together, they can keep out most other little kids. But lectins lock onto the surface of your intestinal cells and flip a switch that makes these tight junctions break apart. It is the equivalent of a playground bully, ramming its way through the junctions between cells, entering the bloodstream and leaving holes in the gut wall that then allow other large molecules, including bacteria, to seep through, creating a condition known as "leaky gut."

Once in the bloodstream, these intestinal escapees trigger an immune response—because the body doesn't recognize them, and it considers them invaders. This fires up inflammation, which explains why so many of my patients have high blood levels of inflammatory cytokines—chemicals that alert the immune system to a threat.

The Lectin Paradox: They Are Both Good *and* Bad

It's so convenient when we can put things in definitive categories—bad guys are evil, good guys are heroes. But when it comes to lectins, they can actually play both roles. Some lectins are inherently beneficial. Have you heard that garlic has healing properties? (It's true, it does.) Its antiviral abilities are thanks to the lectins it contains. Other lectins play a positive role in the body even though they are technically toxic— in small amounts, they educate your immune system about what kinds of compounds are safe and which aren't.

To really wrap your brain around the paradox that plants—and the lectins they contain—can be both good for us and bad for us, it helps to understand the concept of hormesis. This principle tells us that certain compounds that are harmful in large amounts can be beneficial in small doses. In this case, it's not the substance itself that's harmful or not harmful, it's *how much* of it we're exposed to over time that determines its effects. Another way of thinking about it is Paracelsus's observation: "The dose makes the poison."

Hormesis points clearly to one health-promoting strategy, which is to eat a varied diet. That way, you don't rely too much on any one thing. It also explains why our recent shifts to relying more on a few crops for the majority of our caloric intake, primarily wheat, corn, and soy, has made us more susceptible to lectins than our ancestors were. I hope that the recipes in this cookbook and the principles I share in this chapter will help you expand your repertoire to all kinds of foods that you weren't consuming regularly before, whether that's new-to-you, no-lectin grains such as millet and sorghum, or a wider variety of green leafy and cruciferous vegetables. Thanks to hormesis, nature rewards the adventurous palate!

Human Evolution Hasn't Caught Up

Right about now you may well be wondering: if lectins have been around for millions of years, how have humans managed to survive all this time? How could it be that plants are causing us a problem only now?

Well, for one thing, the discovery of fire and subsequent development of cooking about one hundred thousand years ago gave us a leg up over other animals, because cooking breaks down many lectins. Cooking also made it possible for us to start eating tubers, such as yams and sweet potatoes, which are indigestible in their raw state but are, as you probably know, delectable once cooked. The starches from these tubers helped feed our friendly gut bacteria, known as the microbiome, as well as the bacteria that live on the skin and even hover around us, known as the holobiome (kind of like the cloud that follows around the *Peanuts* character, Pig-Pen).

The inhabitants of your microbiome play many important roles in your body, but the two most crucial are that they break down the food you eat and extract nutrients from it and they communicate with your immune system, both alerting it to invaders and doing battle or de-weaponizing harmful substances. Because they are so helpful to us, I call them our "gut buddies."

As our species evolved, so did our gut buddies to handle the lectins in the plants and leaves we consumed. We thrived as a result. When our diet mostly consisted of foraged plants, tubers, and the occasional woolly mammoth steak, we were the picture of health—the average height for males was nearly five feet eleven inches tall (females averaged five foot two).[1]

Then, about ten thousand years ago, the last Ice Age ended and many of the animals and plants that humans relied upon for our main source of calories died off. We had to find new foods to eat. That's when the practice of cultivating crops was born. We started growing grains and beans—two plant foods that were revolutionary because once harvested, they could be stored for later use. While on one hand this was a miraculous feat of ingenuity, it also introduced a whole new array of lectins into our diet; lectins that we weren't equipped to digest, and neither were our bacterial populations.

Ten thousand years may seem like a long enough time for us to evolve a microbiotic population that can handle lectins, but it's not. You have to remember that Mother Nature has a completely different timetable than we do. Even though we can create new technologies (such as fire, agriculture, and wifi) at ever increasing speeds, she needs millennia to adapt to them. In evolutionary terms, ten thousand years is a blink; it's like we've been speed-dating lectins. Our bodies simply weren't prepared to consume them once we started growing our own food, and we still aren't. Is it any wonder that after eating this new diet for two thousand years, the average human height was five feet four inches for males and four feet nine inches for females?[2]

Fast forward to just five hundred years ago, when the "New World"—aka the Americas—was discovered, and our ancestors from Africa, Europe, and Asia were introduced to new, lectin-rich foods they'd never before encountered: tomatoes, squash, corn, chia seeds, quinoa, and other grains. Native American populations, who had been eating these foods for about fifteen to twenty thousand years, may have had the time to develop some specialized gut bugs to digest them. But those new to Western agriculture had no such capacity.

Before they arrived on the shores of the Americas, our ancestors had learned to prepare and preserve foods in ways that, however coincidentally, made them easier to digest. Fermentation is one such method. Traditional cultures have long used fermentation as a means of preserving vegetables and dairy products—think kefir in the Middle East, sauerkraut in Eastern Europe, yogurt in India, kimchi in Korea, or miso in Japan (these are just a handful of examples). Many old world cooking methods also removed the peels, hulls, and seeds from plants, which are the parts that tend to contain the highest concentration of lectins. For example, in Asia, where rice is a staple crop, the hull is typically removed to create white rice. In Europe, where breads and pastas are culinary mainstays, the wheat is similarly stripped of its protective (and lectin-rich) bran and was traditionally eaten only when fresh—a day-old baked good was considered inedible, because when you grind a grain its naturally occurring fats spoil very quickly.

When our ancestors encountered new foods, these traditional preparation methods helped to protect them from consuming harmful amounts of lectins. For more than five hundred years, we continued to use these methods to make our foods more digestible. But in the last one hundred years or so, changes in our culture, food supply, and technology have made us more susceptible to damage from lectins. These changes include:

- Year-round access to fruits and other produce that would otherwise only be available during a short season, meaning we're eating more of these foods that we originally ate only once a year to fatten up for the upcoming winter.

- A disconnection from traditional means of preparing foods (which reduce lectin content) and an overreliance on processed foods that are made primarily from grains and processed oils that are high in lectins.

- An increase in the amount of wheat, corn, and soy we consume—in the form of bread, animal feed (since we essentially end up eating whatever the animals we consume eat), vegetable oil, and processed food.

- Exposure to decades' and millions of dollars' worth of marketing regarding the healthfulness of whole grains and vegetable oils—which are essentially lectin bombs—leaving us woefully confused about which foods actually promote good health. Generations of Americans have loaded up on whole wheat bread and pasta and multigrain bagels thinking that they were making healthy choices— while rates of obesity, diabetes, and heart disease skyrocketed.

So not only have our bodies not yet evolved new gut bugs to deal with new lectins, we're also no longer preparing high-lectin foods in the ways our ancestors did, *and* we're eating more of these foods than ever before. But wait: there's more.

The Seven Deadly Disruptors

Recent developments in the medicine we take and the environment in which we live are also hurting our health. These technological "advances" are actually setting us back in many ways and wreaking havoc on the quantity and diversity of our gut microbes.

I call these modern developments the Seven Deadly Disruptors. I go into great (some might say painstaking) detail about them in *The Plant Paradox*, but for our purposes here I will try to be brief.

1. **BROAD-SPECTRUM ANTIBIOTICS.** While antibiotics can be a life-saving drug, they can also threaten your long-term health by wiping out your supportive bacterial population. We tend to take antibiotics too frequently (you do not need an antibiotic for a cold or the flu!), and we unwittingly consume them every time we eat conventionally raised meat, as most livestock are fed antibiotics to help them stay alive and to fatten them up for slaughter. Think about that: antibiotics are used to fatten animals for slaughter. They do the same to you!

2. **NONSTEROIDAL ANTI-INFLAMMATORY DRUGS (NSAIDS).** Ibuprofen (Advil and Motrin), naproxen (Aleve), Celebrex, and others are popular pain relievers that fall in the category of NSAIDs. NSAIDs damage the lining of the small intestine and colon, which is also targeted by lectins and plays a crucial role in keeping your immune system in good working order. In a cruel cycle, when you regularly take NSAIDs, the damage in your intestinal wall leads to more inflammation, which leads to more pain, which causes you to keep reaching for NSAIDs.

3. **STOMACH-ACID BLOCKERS.** When an animal eats a plant with a lot of lectins— such as unripe fruit, for example—it will get a stomachache and quickly learn to avoid that particular plant in the future. When a human eats something that causes indigestion, we reach for an acid-blocking drug such as Zantac, Prilosec, Nexium, or Protonix. These drugs, most of which are protein pump inhibitors (PPIs), reduce the amount of stomach acid, which may seem like a good thing until you learn that stomach acid is a key way that your body neutralizes harmful bacteria. And the more bad bacteria you have, the less room and resources your good bacteria have. Since your friendly bacteria play such an important role in immunity, it's no coincidence that people who use acid blockers (and have fewer good gut bugs) have three times the likelihood of getting pneumonia than those

who don't. PPIs also inhibit protein digestion, and as you may remember, lectins are plant proteins. So more PPIs also means more lectins on the loose.

4. **ARTIFICIAL SWEETENERS.** No one hates to hear just how damaging artificial sweeteners are more than me—I was a huge Diet Coke addict for years. I drank eight cans a day! Not coincidentally, I was also seventy pounds overweight. The false sweetness doesn't help you lose weight by saving you calories. On the contrary, it decimates your friendly bacterial population[3] and triggers your brain to seek more sweets and store fat for the winter (which is also what eating fruit in the summer will do). And when you have fewer helpful microbes to eat lectins, lectins can wreak more havoc inside your body.

5. **ENDOCRINE DISRUPTORS.** Endocrine disruptors are chemicals that interfere with the normal functioning of your hormones. They are commonly found in plastics, including personal care products, household cleaners, food packaging, cling wrap, food storage containers, and any number of other consumer products. Endocrine disruptors are also found in the food beneath the plastic. Remember how I said that the fats in whole grains quickly spoil once they've been ground? Well, food industry scientists are aware of this and thus add chemical stabilizing agents, such as butylated hydroxytoluene (BHT), to packaged baked goods. BHT is an endocrine disruptor.

No matter where they come from, endocrine disruptors play a role in obesity, many cancers, thyroid problems, and reproductive issues. They also tax your liver—which is the waste treatment plant of your body—and make it harder for it to eliminate excess hormones and to convert vitamin D into its active form. Low levels of vitamin D are associated with numerous diseases, including autoimmune diseases, dementia, Alzheimer's, heart disease, osteoporosis, breast cancer, and prostate cancer. Moreover, vitamin D helps to keep the wall of your gut intact in the battle with lectins. Less vitamin D, more lectins, more "leaky gut."

6. **GENETICALLY MODIFIED FOODS AND THE HERBICIDE ROUNDUP.** Most genetically modified foods have been bred to withstand the pesticide known as glyphosate, the main ingredient in Roundup, a pesticide made by Monsanto and Enlist, which is manufactured by Dow Chemical. Because the GMO plants don't die when exposed to glyphosate, farmers can douse their fields with the stuff and the main crop—generally wheat, corn, or soy—won't die. But here's what you probably didn't know: Roundup is now used on non-GMO versions of these same plants as a desiccant, because a dried-up, dead plant is easier to harvest. This practice is particularly common with oats, grains, legumes, and beans, which means it's incredibly important to choose organic versions of these foods

(if you choose to eat them at all; following the Plant Paradox guidelines will help you avoid many of these foods, but keep it in mind if you continue to eat beans—preferably beans that have been pressure-cooked to destroy their lectins, something I'll cover more in Chapter 2). These chemicals are passed along to who- or whatever eats the crop, whether it's you, your kids, or the animals that eventually show up on your dinner table. This means you get a dose of Roundup even if you meticulously avoid GMO foods but eat either nonorganic grains or meat that was fed nonorganic grains. In addition to being classified as a probable human carcinogen by the World Health Organization[4] (although different divisions of the organization disagree on this assessment,[5] and a study published in November 2017, found no increased incidence of cancer in farm workers who handled glyphosate[6]) and found to contribute to fatty liver disease at low doses in rats,[7] Roundup also depletes your friendly gut bacteria.

7. **BLUE LIGHT.** Your body is exquisitely designed to take its cues for fat storage and fat burning from its daily exposure to light. When days are long and nights are short (in summer), we are cued to store fat in preparation for the coming winter, when food was typically scarce. And when days are short and nights are long, our body gets a signal to burn its own fat stores since calories from food were generally reduced. Now, we stare at electronic devices all day that emit blue light—the part of the light spectrum that comprises daylight—making our internal clocks think it's summer all the time. As a result, we are continually getting the message to store fat and to seek out more calories.

Lectins and Autoimmunity

Your digestive tract is a sealed tube that starts at your mouth, goes down your throat, and coils around in your abdomen, leading to your anus. Any food particles that enter that tube aren't technically part of your body—they stay in the tube. It's like a tunnel that goes through a river; you travel in that tunnel, you are surrounded by water but you don't get wet because you aren't actually *in* the river.

All food you consume travels down the throat, through the esophagus, into the stomach, and eventually makes its way to your intestines to be transformed into tiny molecules of nutrients that your body can use or excrete as waste. If you stretched out your intestines, they would cover the surface area of a tennis court. However, the width of the intestinal wall—which is all that separates the food you eat from your bloodstream—is only one cell thick, and these cells normally have an impenetrable seal between them. Your intestinal wall is designed to let single molecules of digested food, individual amino acids, fatty acids, and sugars pass from inside your gut to your bloodstream—that's it. In order to shore up the gut wall, your body produces a mucous barrier on the inside of it, and that mucus is made of up polysaccharides, which are a form of sugar.

When you eat lectins, remember, they are looking for sugar molecules to attach to. So what do they do? They bind to the sugar molecules in the mucosal lining of your intestines. Once there, they trigger the production of zonulin, which is a protein that serves as a key to open those tight junctions between the cells of your gut wall. When your cells produce zonulin, they stop linking arms, and any lectins that haven't yet bound to the mucus lining seep out of the tunnel and into the bloodstream, bringing with them pieces of bacteria called lipopolysaccharides, or LPS for short. I don't normally swear, but I can't resist calling them "little pieces of shit," because that's what they are. Literally. This phenomenon is known as leaky gut syndrome, and it's where lectins become really destructive.

On the other side of that wall is your immune system. Think of your immune system like a border patrol. When the immune system comes in contact with any foreign substance, it sounds the alarm: *The wall has been breached! We're under attack! Prepare for war! Stockpile supplies and assemble the army!* The supplies in this case are fat cells, the army is made up of white blood cells, and the weapon this army uses is inflammation. This is why the body stores fat wherever a war is being waged. And when the war is in your gut, the result is abdominal fat—which Dr. William Davis made famous as a "wheat belly." Even worse, though, when the immune system remains continually in war mode, what is a healthy response can easily cross over into full-on autoimmune disease, which is what happens when the immune system attacks healthy cells of the body that aren't dangerous or invaders. Common autoimmune diseases include rheumatoid arthritis, Crohn's disease, lupus, Hashimoto's disease, MS, Grave's disease, celiac disease, vitiligo, psoriasis, IBS, and type 1 diabetes. In my practice, I have seen patients resolve their autoimmune issues simply by removing lectins from their diet. That's because by avoiding or neutralizing lectins in your food, you remove a root cause of autoimmunity and give your gut and your microbiome a chance to heal.

In a fascinating paper published in 2017 in the *Journal of Diabetes Research*,[8] researchers from Harvard Medical School and Loma Linda University School of Medicine tested the autoimmune response of pancreatic islet cells in the presence of a number of different foods, all of which are on the low-glycemic diet recommended to diabetic patients. The vast majority of foods they found to provoke an autoimmune response are high in lectins, including cow's milk, non-gluten grains such as buckwheat and oats, lentils, peas, and chickpeas. Interestingly, seaweed, pecans, and goat's milk also triggered significant responses, and wheat—which contains gluten—didn't score as high as many non-gluten grains. While the paper doesn't prove causation between eating these foods and type 1 diabetes (the form of the disease with an autoimmune component), it does show that many lectin-rich foods are associated with an autoimmune response in the pancreatic cells that become damaged and contribute to type 1 diabetes, suggesting that we need to revamp our food recommendations for diabetics. But why wait until you or your child has developed type 1 diabetes to remove a known autoimmunity trigger from your diet?

How Lectins Cause Weight Gain

As we've just discussed, eating high-lectin foods like wheat cues your body to store fat because the lectins they contain wage war on your gut, and the troops need food (aka stored fat) to keep battling. And as we know from our discussion of the microbiome, lectins also deplete beneficial gut microbes, which support our well-being in a number of important ways—including helping to maintain a healthy weight.

But there's also a third reason why eating lectin-rich foods contributes to excess weight: because one of the lectins in many grains (in addition to gluten) is wheat germ agglutinin (WGA), which is one of the most offensive lectins out there and has been implicated in celiac disease and heart disease. One of its (as well as other lectins') most insidious powers, however, is that it has the ability to mimic insulin in the body.

Insulin is a hormone that's manufactured by the pancreas, which releases varying amounts of it in response to the amount of sugar and protein you eat. Insulin helps regulate your blood sugar levels by attaching to either fat cells, nerve cells (or neurons), or muscle cells and ordering them to open up and let the glucose in. Once the glucose is moved into the cell, the insulin detaches and these cells are able to receive messages from other hormones and chemical messengers.

But WGA binds to the same receptor sites on these cell walls that insulin does. And it doesn't ever leave. So the next time your gut releases glucose into your bloodstream, the insulin doesn't have a place to attach to. It's kind of like insulin is you in your car and the cell wall is the grocery store parking lot. If all the parking spaces are filled with other cars, and no one ever leaves, you can never park and actually go into the store to get the food you need.

When WGA attaches to your fat cells, it can stay there indefinitely as well, continually telling them to make more fat from the sugar that passes by. When it parks on the wall of a muscle cell, it prevents any sugar cells from getting in. As a result, your muscle cell can't access the fuel it needs to maintain itself and grow; muscle wasting is the outcome. And when lectins take up residence on insulin receptors on nerve cells, your neurons never get the energy that they need, and so they continually send a message that you're hungry in hopes of getting more fuel. So your nervous system keeps sending hunger signals, even when you've had plenty of calories. The sum result of WGA mimicking insulin is that your fat cells grow, your calorie consumption rises, your brain cells don't get the fuel they need (leading to brain fog), and muscle tone reduces. Does any of this sound familiar?

The Road Back to Good Health

The good news is that once you understand what lectins are and where they come from, it is possible to settle into a way of eating that has cascading positive effects on health—from troubling symptoms like bloating and brain fog up to outright disease such as heart disease and autoimmune disease.

Even better, as I will show you in the chapters to come, these foods that are so good for your immune system and supportive of your friendly gut bacteria population are also delicious. Whether or not you follow the full Plant Paradox plan (which I will outline in Chapter 2), you'll find recipes here for foods that satisfy your inner gut buddies *and* your taste buds.

chapter two

"So What Exactly Can I Eat?!"

After people read *The Plant Paradox*, one of the most common reactions I get is "What's left for me to eat??"

I promise you, I am not out to deprive you of the foods you love—that's why I wrote this cookbook.

There are some foods that I will suggest you stop eating altogether, and yes, that will be an adjustment, but I'm going to go out on a limb here and wager that you weren't really enjoying some of them—like whole wheat bread and brown rice—to begin with.

The great news is that many of your favorite high-lectin foods can be cooked or prepared in such a way to reduce their lectin content. So no, you don't have to give up beans or tomatoes for the rest of your life, but you can make it easier on your gut and your immune system by preparing them a little differently.

I do want to be clear about one thing: There is no way to eliminate every single lectin from your diet, nor would I suggest you try to do so. In fact, not all lectins are troublesome—plants have been creating these chemical compounds for millions of years, and some of them do foster human health, particularly those contained in plants we've been eating for millennia. For some of my "canaries"—the patients in my practice who show higher-than-average sensitivity to lectins—small amounts of certain lectins are enough to trigger severe reactions. But other patients of mine consumed large quantities of lectin-containing foods for years without noticing an effect.

Remember, our bodies don't adapt to new conditions, or new foods, overnight. Our microbiomes and our immune system have had ample time to adjust to the lectins and other compounds contained in the plants we've been eating for millennia (such as those on the "yes, please" list on the following pages). It's the "newer" foods—those we've only been eating for about ten thousand years—that are the most problematic for our physiologies. These foods include grains and beans and New World plants like corn and tomatoes. So while it's impossible to avoid *all* lectins, you can radically improve your health by controlling which ones you consume and how much of them you eat. Like the line in the 1956 movie *The Court Jester*, "The pellet with the poison's in the flagon with the dragon; the vessel with the pestle has the brew that is true," I just want to give you a guide to where the poisons are lurking.

Let's start with the brew that is true.

Yes, Please: Foods That Are Low in Lectins

GOOD FATS

Generally, I advise that anywhere between 60 and 80 percent of your total daily calories come from healthy fat sources. I know—that sounds like an awful lot of fat! Especially in light of all the misguided nutritional advice we've been fed (pardon the pun) for years about fat being bad for us. Some fat is bad for us, but not all fat is created equal. While there are many oils that I don't recommend consuming, such as those made from high-lectin vegetable seeds, good quality fats are essential for your health.

Believe it or not, eating fat can actually help you lose weight. Healthy fats don't contain glucose (which gets stored as fat when you eat too much of it) or trigger the release of insulin (which tells the body to store excess glucose as fat) like carbohydrates do. Some types of fat also help to protect and nourish the cells of your gut lining.[9] In addition, your brain is comprised of 60 percent fat, so eating healthy fat also feeds your brain. **The best sources of healthy fats are extra-virgin olive oil, olives, avocados, avocado oil, coconut milk, MCT oil (otherwise known as medium-chain triglyceride oil or liquid coconut oil), coconut oil, perilla oil, walnut oil, macadamia oil, algae oil, egg yolks from pastured chicken, and most importantly, fish oil or algae-based DHA.** These foods, along with leafy greens and cruciferous vegetables, should form the foundation of your daily food intake.

GREENS

Green leafy vegetables are so good for you it's nearly impossible to eat more than you need; nearly everyone's diet is lacking in greens. These plants are high in chemicals called polyphenols that support full-body health. Where lectins protect their host plants by causing harm to any creatures that consume the plant, polyphenols make the plants themselves stronger. And so, when we eat polyphenols, they lend us some of their restorative powers. Beyond the polyphenols that greens provide, they are very filling, especially when combined with a healthy fat, like a generous covering of olive or avocado oil. Meaning, eating more greens will naturally reduce any cravings for less healthful foods. In fact, you'll find that you start craving greens instead!

Good sources of greens include lettuce (romaine, butter, red, and green leaf), dandelion greens, mesclun, spinach, endive, parsley, mustard greens, fennel, and seaweed/sea vegetables.

CRUCIFEROUS VEGETABLES AND LECTIN-FREE VEGETABLES

Vegetables are excellent sources of prebiotic fiber, vitamins, and polyphenols, and should comprise the majority of your meals. Cruciferous vegetables are especially nutritious and offer a number of health benefits. They activate specialized white blood cells in the lining of your gut, and those cells have the ability to tell an overactive immune system to stand down. Since eating a high-lectin diet has likely irritated your gut wall and prompted your immune system into a hyper-aroused state, cruciferous veggies are just the thing to help restore your gut health. **Good choices include broccoli, cabbage, cauliflower, kale, Brussels sprouts, collard greens, Swiss chard, bok choy, watercress, kohlrabi, and arugula.** And don't neglect other lectin-free veggies such as **artichokes, asparagus, garlic, celery, leeks, radishes, beets, mushrooms, okra, and onions**—they will fill you up and deliver a tasty cocktail of nutrients!

NUTS

Nuts are a great source of healthy fats, polyphenols, and fiber, and are okay to eat every day, but in limited amounts (because their caloric and protein content can add up quickly). They make fabulous snacks because they are portable (it's easy to keep a stash in your desk drawer or glove box) and filling. It's important to note, however, that not every nut is compatible with the Plant Paradox program. Legumes like peanuts and cashews should be avoided. **I recommend sticking to macadamias, walnuts, pistachios, pecans, coconuts, hazelnuts, and chestnuts.** Some nuts can also be used as flour alternatives—your best bets are coconut flour or almond flour. Everyone asks about almonds. The skin or peel of almonds have a lectin that many of my autoimmune patients react to; blanched or Marcona almonds are peeled and seem to be safe. That's why blanched almond flour makes the list and almonds do not.

AVOCADOS

Yes, we covered avocados in the "Good Fats" section just a few paragraphs earlier in this section, but it's such a nutritional superstar and so readily available that it's worth calling out on its own. Avocados are full of good fat and soluble fiber, both of which are key to helping you lose weight and absorb polyphenols (many plant-based vitamins are fat soluble, meaning you need to eat them with a fat in order to reap their benefits). Avocados contain heart-healthy monounsaturated fat, just like olive oil. In fact, eating an avocado a day has been shown to reduce LDL cholesterol—the dangerous kind of cholesterol—by 13.5 mg/dl.[10] That's a significant amount for one easy dietary change! Now, avocado is a fruit, but it's actually okay to eat when ripe because it's essentially sugar-free. You're already accustomed to the idea that eating one piece of fruit every day—namely, an apple—can keep the doctor away. Just replace that apple with an avocado and you will be well on your way to promoting a healthy heart and a healthy weight.

LECTIN-FREE GRAINS

I know it's challenging to think about giving up all grains—not only are they incredibly convenient because they are ubiquitous, they're also probably what you've come to consider as your go-to foods. Sandwiches, granola bars, wraps, cereal—grains are some of the easiest convenience foods, and they're often marketed to us as "health foods." Nothing could be further from the truth!

But there are a couple of grains that don't contain lectins—sorghum and millet, to be exact. Sorghum is an awesome lectin-free, gluten-free flour alternative that's chock full of fiber. It also contains chemical compounds that have been shown to be beneficial to friendly gut bacteria and positively impact obesity, diabetes, and inflammation in animals and in in vitro lab tests.[11] Millet is packed with important minerals like magnesium, potassium, phosphorus, and zinc. Not only that, the polyphenols in millet offer more health benefits than most grains.[12] If you're wondering how to prepare and serve these grains, check out the recipes for my Sorghum Bowl (page 153), Moroccan-Spiced Chicken with Millet Tabbouleh (page 178), and Thanksgiving Millet Stuffing (page 200).

RESISTANT STARCHES

Resistant starches are carbohydrates that give you a (mostly) free pass when it comes to their caloric content and impact on blood sugar levels. When you eat a typical carbohydrate, such as a piece of bread or bowl of rice, your body quickly converts it to glucose, which is then either burned for energy or stored as fat. A resistant starch, on the other hand, does not get broken down and converted into glucose quickly—and much of it passes through your small intestine intact. This is because these starches aren't susceptible to the enzymes that break down regular starches; that's why they're called "resistant." While *you* can't digest resistant starches, your friendly gut bacteria can. They proliferate on a diet of resistant starches and crowd out the bad bugs that also live in your digestive tract.[13] In addition, your gut buddies convert resistant starches to short-chain fatty acids, many of which are a preferred form of fuel for your colon and your neurons, even the neurons in your far-away brain.

Sweet potatoes, yams, yucca, green plantains, cassava, tapioca, green bananas, jicama, and taro root are all resistant starches as well as great sources of vitamins and minerals. That's because these tubers have roots with strong absorption abilities that draw water and minerals from the soil for nourishment. Also, they're high in fiber, which is a source of fuel for your gut bugs. It's okay to eat resistant starches every day, just try to eat them in moderation and limit the quantity with each meal. Over years of tracking thousands of patients and their eating habits and blood work, I've noticed that some of my overzealous resistant-starch eaters start to gain excess weight. I mean, who wouldn't gain weight eating three big plantain pancakes three times a day with a sweet potato as a side dish?

WILD-CAUGHT SEAFOOD

Fish and shellfish are some of the healthiest and tastiest foods out there. Seafood is a great source of protein and provides vitamin D and omega-3 fatty acids, which have numerous benefits, including reducing inflammation,[14] protecting against heart disease,[15] and boosting brain health.

The thing is, you want to make sure the seafood that ends up on your plate is wild-caught and not farm-raised, even if it is labeled organic. Among other things, farm-raised fish, because of the crowded conditions, are often treated with antibiotics or even treated with pesticides and fed corn and soy (both of which are full of lectins), whereas wild-caught fish have eaten a natural diet. Please don't be misled by the organic label on salmon or other fish. The organic label means they were fed organic grains and soy. Do you really think they followed the salmon around the ocean to see that they ate "organically"? My wife and I tend to eat mostly vegetarian or vegan during the week, but on the weekends we have a serving of wild seafood each day, for variety and for taste. I call our approach to eating "Vegaquarian."

PASTURED POULTRY AND OMEGA-3 EGGS

Pastured poultry can be a great source of protein and, if you eat the yolks of your eggs or the skin on your chicken, fat. But pastured is not the same thing as free-range or organic. Often, free-range chickens are never shown the light of day. And they're fed corn and soy. **So the only type of poultry I recommend you eat is pastured.** These are chickens that have been allowed to roam and forage for their food—as insectivores, their natural diet is grubs and other insects. Look for the words "pasture-raised" or "pastured" on the label of the chickens, or talk to the farmers at your local farmer's market and ask how their chickens are fed. (I asked this question of a farmer at my local market in Santa Barbara, and she said, "I don't feed my chickens anything, they work for me!" Meaning they fed themselves lots of tasty bugs.)

When it comes to eggs, I recommend purchasing either pastured eggs (meaning eggs from chickens that were allowed to roam and forage for their food) or omega-3 eggs (eggs you can purchase at most grocery stores that say "omega-3" somewhere on the label). As we've just discussed, omega-3 acids are important for your health, and research shows omega-3 eggs can help lower cholesterol.[16] And believe it or not, I want you to eat the yolks and limit the whites! Yes, exactly the opposite of the "yolks are bad for you" old dietary advice. Try a four-yolk, one-egg-white omelet and give the other egg whites to your dog or cat.

One-hundred Percent Grass-fed Meat

Let's pause for a moment to celebrate: You can have meat! But it must be specific kind of meat: grass-fed and pasture-raised. Why are these designations important? Remember, you are what the thing you are eating ate. If you eat meat from animals that were fed corn and soy, you are essentially eating lectin-rich corn and soy, much of which has been genetically modified to contain even more lectins than unadulterated strains of the same plants. Moreover, most grains and soy are now sprayed with Roundup, which makes its way into the meats of these animals and therefore into you.

So when you eat meat, absolutely make sure it was grass-fed and grass-finished. The meat from these animals contains more omega-3 and fewer omega-6 fats, which are easily oxidized and thus inflammatory, than animals raised on conventional feed lots. **Suitable choices include bison,**

Deciphering the Labels on Poultry, Eggs, and Meat

Because you end up consuming whatever the animals you eat consumed, you want to be choosy when selecting the chickens, eggs, and meats you buy at the store. Unfortunately, the labels on these food items are confusing and sometimes downright misleading. This chart can help you determine what each designation means, so you can choose the animal product that best serves your needs for nutrition.

WHEN THE LABEL SAYS...	IT MEANS...
ORGANIC	When it comes to meat, poultry, and eggs, the organic designation means the animals aren't fed growth hormones or antibiotics, they are fed organic feed (meaning no GMOs or chemical pesticides or fertilizers used to grow the grains and soy used for feed), and they must have outdoor access. "Organic" is the only label that requires government inspection and verification. It's a good label to look for when buying meat, but the very best label is "pastured" or "grass-fed and -finished." This is because grains and soy are not a natural diet for chickens (who eat insects) or for cows (who eat grasses) or other animals raised for meat, meaning even an organic diet is nutritionally lacking for animals.
ALL VEGETARIAN-FED	Found mostly on poultry products, this means the chickens weren't fed animal by-products. Which likely means that they were given feed that contains grains, pseudo-grains, and/or soy, most of which are loaded with lectins and GMO. Beyond that, chickens are natural insect-eaters, so a vegetarian diet isn't actually all that healthy for them!
FREE RANGE	This designation, as codified in a 2007 federal law, means that animals are given access to the outside for at least five minutes a day. Free-range chickens typically still live in a crowded barn that has some sort of opening—no matter how small—to the outside. This outside can be a small, muddy, fenced-in or netted-in yard, and the barn may be so crowded that most chickens never make it out.
CAGE FREE	Though it may conjure images of chickens freely roaming around a grass field, cage-free means that the chickens aren't confined to cages—but they are still likely to be confined to an overcrowded barn with no guarantee of ever going outside.

WHEN THE LABEL SAYS...	IT MEANS...
PASTURE-RAISED	"Pasture-raised" hens have to be limited to 1,000 birds for every 2.5 acres. That's 108 sq. ft. per bird—approximately 106 sq. ft. more per bird than required for the "free range" designation. Field rotation is mandatory, meaning the hens have to get continual access to grassy fields, not the same area that has already been picked over day and after day by the flock. Also, the hens must be kept outdoors throughout the year—with safe, accessible housing should the hens need to protect themselves from predators, or shelter themselves from extreme weather. When it comes to chicken, pasture-raised really is the highest standard possible.
OMEGA-3	You'll see this term on some egg cartons—it means the eggs were laid by hens who consume a natural diet enhanced with flaxseed and/or algae. When the flax and algae is digested, the polyunsaturated omega-3 fatty acid gets transferred to the yolk. In a recent study, omega-3 eggs had approximately five times as much omega-3 fatty acid as conventional eggs.[17] Although these chickens likely aren't allowed to forage for their natural diet of grasses and insects and whatever else they can pick out of a patch of dirt, omega-3 eggs are often your best alternative if you can't find eggs from chickens that were pasture-raised.
HORMONE-FREE	You'll see this term on egg cartons as well as labels of poultry and meat. It simply means the animals weren't administered any hormones. It doesn't mean they weren't fed lectin-rich or GMO grains or animal by-products, or given antibiotics.
ANTIBIOTIC-FREE	Similar to the "hormone-free" designation, this means only that the animals didn't get antibiotic injections or have antibiotics added to their feed. It doesn't mean they were fed a natural diet or that they weren't given hormones.
GRASS-FED	Generally used in relation to beef and other animals raised for beef, this designation only means the animals were given access to grass at some point in their lives. Animals raised for meat are often given hay and access to grass for a little while, then fattened up for slaughter on a diet of grains, antibiotics, and growth hormones. That's why you want to look for meat that either says "grass-fed and grass-finished" or "100 percent grass-fed," because these mean the animals ate their natural diet for their whole life.

wild game, venison, boar, elk, pork (humanely raised), lamb, beef, and prosciutto di Parma. But, like dairy, moderation is key, because all of this meat contains a specific sugar molecule, Neu5Gc, which is associated with cancer and heart disease. Ideally, you'll keep your consumption of animal protein to four ounces or less per day, and certainly no more than eight ounces (and don't even think about a twenty-four-ounce porterhouse!). We'll talk about other reasons to limit your animal protein intake a little bit later in this chapter.

IN-SEASON FRUITS

Fruit is a good source of fiber, vitamins, and polyphenols, but you must be very mindful of how much you eat and when you eat it. First of all, because it contains so much sugar, think of it more like candy than a "health food" and eat it sparingly. In addition, the fruit must be—I repeat, *must be*—in season. Turns out, eating fruit in season was a great thing for our ancestors, because it allowed them to fatten up for the winter months. But now, we can get fruit anytime—and thus, send the signal to our bodies that we need to store fat all year long. (If you're interested, I go into significant detail as to why in-season fruits should be viewed as a treat in *The Plant Paradox*.)

There are a few fruits that are great to eat year-round. The only hitch is, they've got to be eaten while they're still green. They include bananas, mangoes, and papayas.

These fruits are okay to consume year-round because when unripe, they've not yet expanded their sugar content. And the good bacteria in our guts love to feast on the perfect prebiotic fibers they contain.

Want the benefit of fruit without the sugar? Bring your juicer out of storage, juice your fruits and berries, throw the juice away (or give it to your friend who's on a "juice cleanse"), and use the pulp! Mix it with coconut or goat yogurt, or add it to a smoothie of greens and protein.

SPECIFIC TYPES OF DAIRY

Nearly all of the cow's milk dairy available in the United States and Canada comes from breeds of cows (including Holstein, the most common breed of cow worldwide) that produce a lectin-like protein known as casein A1. **The good news is that milk from goats, sheep, and water buffalo (as well as milk from Guernsey, Brown Swiss, and Belgian Blue breeds of cows,** although these cows are rare in North America) does not contain this protein and so can be enjoyed on the Plant Paradox program.

As it turns out, casein A1 is converted to protein called beta-casomorphin, which can prompt an autoimmune attack on the human pancreas when consumed.[18] This is then believed to cause some serious health concerns, such as type 1 diabetes.

So, stick to Southern European cow's milk, goat's milk, sheep's milk, and buffalo milk and the cheeses made from these milks. Health food stores are pretty good about carrying these (I recommend specific brands in the recipe section). Also, consider these milks an indulgence and consume them only in moderate quantities, as they do contain Neu5Gc.

CHOCOLATE AND APPROVED ALCOHOL

Cocoa or specifically cacao, the primary ingredient in chocolate, is an undeniable health food—it contains polyphenols, flavonoids, and fiber, all of which have anti-inflammatory properties. Chocolate is also known to be heart healthy: the *British Medical Journal* published a study offering evidence that eating chocolate may reduce the risk of cardiovascular disease by up to one third![19] Just as importantly, it is delicious and can really soothe cravings for something sweet. The problem is that the sugar and dairy products that are often added to cocoa to make commercial chocolates not all that good for you, and they tend to be highly caloric as well, which leads to weight gain. In order to get the benefits of chocolate without incurring the downsides, **eat dark chocolate—72 percent cocoa or higher—and limit yourself to one ounce a day or less.**

Consuming red wine in moderation can actually help your health—studies have shown that the polyphenols in red wine might be connected to reduced risk of cardiovascular disease and other heart health issues.[20] **Limit wine consumption to one four-to-six-ounce glass a day, only during meals.** When drinking red wine, choose cool-climate pinot noirs such as Oregonian wines or red wines from high elevations such as an Argentinian malbec or Chilean cabernet. Why? Chilly weather and high elevations are good for producing high concentrations of resveratrol—a powerful polyphenol. If you do buy Argentinian or Chilean wines, make sure to buy organic and/or biodynamic. (Wine from these countries is usually high in pesticides due to lack of regulation.) Avoid white wine, as it tends to have more sugar and lacks the powerful polyphenols—namely, resveratrol and quercetin—contained in red wine.

Also, if you're going to drink liquor, choose a dark spirit, such as whisky, that has been aged in a wood barrel. Why? The wood in the barrels contains polyphenols that are then absorbed into the spirit. Avoid clear spirits, such as vodka.

And if you really want to be festive, opt for a glass of champagne. The grapes that go into champagne contain important polyphenols that potentially improve memory.[21] Again, all these alcoholic beverages should be consumed in very moderate amounts.

Just Say No: Foods High in Lectins

The Plant Paradox program is based on this essential truth: The foods you don't eat are far more important to your health than the foods you do eat.

We will discuss this idea in more detail in Chapter 3, but the basic premise of the Plant Paradox program is that once you remove the inflammatory agents (aka lectins) from your diet, your body is able to stop throwing all its resources and energy into dealing with continual damage and go into restorative mode, where excess weight can be released and diseases can be healed.

To that end, here are the basic categories of foods that are excluded from the Plant Paradox program. These are foods that no human ate until about ten thousand years ago—and today we are still woefully ill-equipped to digest them.

I've compiled all of these "yes, please" and "no, thank you" foods into a much handier list, which appears on pages 29–32. You'll notice the list of "yes, please" foods is more than twice as long as the list of "no, thank you" foods. But because knowing the reason *why* a food should be avoided will help empower you to consistently choose not to eat it. Let's chat briefly about what makes these food off-limits.

PEANUTS AND CASHEWS

Despite the fact that you probably think of these two popular foods as nuts, they are not. They are legumes, and as such are loaded with killer lectins. In fact, the shell that sheaths a cashew is so caustic that workers must wear protective gloves to shell them! In my medical practice, I have witnessed first-hand that eating cashews dramatically increases inflammation, especially in patients with rheumatoid arthritis. The cashew is part of the same family as poison ivy; I doubt if you'd consider munching on that. There are plenty of tasty nuts on the "yes, please" list—stick to those and your body will thank you. And if you are a die-hard peanut butter fan, rest assured that its tastier cousin, almond butter, is part of the Plant Paradox program.

CORN

Like nearly all other grains, corn (which is not a vegetable, but a grain) has a high lectin content. And since corn is one of the biggest crops and most common food additives—think corn syrup, cornstarch, corn flakes and other breakfast cereals, corn chips—the typical American eats some form of corn multiple times a day.

QUINOA

This New World pseudo-grain is hailed as a gluten-free substitute to wheat, but it is so loaded with lectins that it is no friend to your digestive tract, immune system, or waistline. Ancient Incas, who made quinoa part of their diet, first soaked it and then fermented it before cooking in an effort to reduce its potential toxicity—two instructions you'll rarely ever see on the side of a box of quinoa.

CONVENTIONALLY RAISED MEAT

It's not difficult to see why corn is among the worst lectin-filled grains. Just look at the American farm industry. Farmers use corn for the sole purpose of fattening up cattle. And, guess what? Corn has the same effect on us. Not only that, it causes fatty deposits in the muscle. So, avoid "free-range" meats and chicken. "Free-range" means the cattle and chicken are eating corn and, therefore, so are you. Instead, opt for only pasture-raised meats and chicken.

VEGETABLE OILS

You may have heard that vegetable oils are healthier for you than other oils, but most of them are made from high-lectin beans or seeds: corn oil, soybean oil, and sunflower oil are all potent sources of lectins. Worse, much of the corn and the soybeans used to make this oil are genetically modified, meaning they have been bred to produce extra-strength lectins that help make them more resistant to insects. On top of this, the fats in these vegetable oils are primarily omega-6 fats, meaning these oils deliver a double-dose of inflammation when you consume them. Finally, I'll say it again, all these oils come from grains or seeds sprayed with Roundup, so it too ends up in you!

LEGUMES AND BEANS

Beans, peas, soybeans, lentils, and other legumes (also known as pulses) have the highest lectin content of any food group. Is it any wonder that they are also renowned for their ability to cause gas, bloating, and indigestion?! I know, I know—beans have been hailed as a mainstay of a healthy diet for decades now, particularly if you eat a vegan or vegetarian diet. Don't get me wrong, I am not against grains and beans! I'm just against eating them without first taming their inflammatory effects. You can dramatically reduce the lectin content of beans and legumes by pressure-cooking them.

DAIRY

Dairy products made from the milk of most North American cows—even those that are grass-fed and organically raised—contain the lectin-like protein casein A1. The only approved dairy products on this plan are those outlined on page 30, which include products made from goat, sheep, and water buffalo milk as well as cow's milk from Southern European cows. The good news here is that coconut milk—the kind that comes in a can as well as the kind that comes in a carton as a milk alternative—makes a great substitute for that creamy dairy taste in soups, ice creams, and other foods.

NIGHTSHADES

This popular family of plants includes potatoes, peppers (bell as well as hot peppers like chili and jalapeño), eggplants, goji berries, and tomatoes—all of which contain a heaping helping of lectins, in addition to the glycoalkoid poison solanine, a known neurotoxin.[22] They are all high in lectins, particularly in their seeds and peels, and therefore unfriendly to your health.

SQUASHES

With the exception of cucumbers, which first originated in Asia and then made their way to Africa and Europe via trade routes, the squash family—fruits with peels and seeds that grow on vines, including pumpkins, acorn squash, zucchini, and butternut squash—is native to the Americas. Meaning, it contains lectins that humans have only been exposed to in the last five hundred years or so. In addition to containing lectins, all varieties of squash contain sugars that cue your body to store weight in preparation for winter. All the more reason not to eat them, or their seeds!

Say "Yes, Please" to These Acceptable Foods

OILS

algae oil (Thrive culinary brand)

olive oil

coconut oil

macadamia oil

MCT oil

avocado oil

perilla oil

walnut oil

red palm oil

rice bran oil

sesame oil

flavored cod liver oil

SWEETENERS

Stevia (SweetLeaf is my favorite)

Just Like Sugar (made from chicory root (inulin))

inulin

yacón (Super Yacon Syrup is available at Walmart, or you can find Sunfood Sweet Yacon Syrup on Amazon)

monk fruit, also known as luo han guo (see below)

luo han guo (the Nutresse brand is good)

erythritol (Swerve is my favorite as it also contains oligosaccharides)

xylitol

NUTS AND SEEDS
(½ cup per day)

macadamia nuts

walnuts

pistachios

pecans

coconuts (not coconut water)

coconut milk (unsweetened dairy substitute)

coconut milk/cream (unsweetened, full-fat, canned)

hazelnuts

chestnuts

brazil nuts (in limited amounts)

pine nuts (in limited amounts)

flax seeds

hemp seeds

hemp protein powder

psyllium

OLIVES

all

DARK CHOCOLATE

72 percent or greater (1 ounce per day)

VINEGARS

all (without added sugar)

HERBS AND SEASONINGS

all except chili pepper flakes

miso

ENERGY BARS

Quest bars: Lemon Cream Pie, Banana Nut, Strawberry Cheesecake, Cinnamon Roll, and Double Chocolate Chunk only

B-Up bars (sometimes found as Yup bars): Chocolate Mint, Chocolate Chip, Cookie Dough, and Sugar Cookie only

Human Food bar

Adapt bar: Coconut and Chocolate (adaptyourlife.com)

FLOURS

coconut

almond

hazelnut

sesame (and seeds)

chestnut

cassava

green banana

sweet potato

tiger nut

grape seed

arrowroot

"FOODLES" (my name for acceptable noodles)

Cappelo's fettucine and other pasta

Pasta Slim

shirataki noodles

kelp noodles

Miracle Noodles and Kanten Pasta

Miracle Rice

Korean sweet potato noodles

(continued)

DAIRY PRODUCTS
(1 ounce cheese or 4 ounces yogurt per day)

Parmigiano-Reggiano

French/Italian butter

buffalo butter (available at Trader Joe's)

ghee

goat yogurt (plain)

goat milk as creamer

goat cheese

butter

goat and sheep kefir (plain)

sheep cheese and yogurt (plain)

coconut yogurt

French/Italian cheese

cheese from Switzerland

buffalo mozzarella (Italy)

whey protein powder

casein A2 milk (as creamer only)

organic heavy cream

organic sour cream

organic cream cheese

ICE CREAM

coconut milk dairy-free frozen desserts (the So Delicious blue label, which contains only 1 gram of sugar)

LaLoo's goat milk ice cream

ALCOHOLIC BEVERAGES

red wine (6 ounces per day)

dark spirits (1 ounce per day)

FISH
(any wild-caught, 4 ounces per day)

whitefish

freshwater bass

Alaskan halibut

canned tuna

Alaskan salmon

Hawaiian fish

shrimp

crab

lobster

scallops

calamari/squid

clams

oysters

mussels

sardines

anchovies

FRUITS (limit all but avocado to one small serving per meal and only when that fruit is in season)

avocados

blueberries

raspberries

blackberries

strawberries

cherries

crispy pears (Anjou, Bosc, Comice)

pomegranates

kiwis

apples

citrus (no juices)

nectarines

passionfruit

peaches

plums

apricots

figs

dates

VEGETABLES

CRUCIFEROUS VEGETABLES

broccoli

Brussels sprouts

cauliflower

bok choy

napa cabbage

Swiss chard

arugula

watercress

collards

kohlrabi

kale

green and red cabbage

radicchio

raw sauerkraut

kimchi

OTHER VEGETABLES

Nopales cactus

celery

onions

leeks

chives

scallions

chicory

carrots (raw)

carrot greens

artichokes

beets (raw)

radishes

daikon radish

Jerusalem artichokes/sunchokes

hearts of palm

cilantro

okra

asparagus

garlic

mushrooms

LEAFY GREENS

romaine

red and green leaf lettuce

mesclun (baby greens)

spinach

endive

dandelion greens

butter lettuce

fennel

escarole

mustard greens

mizuna

parsley

basil

mint

purslane

perilla

algae

seaweed

sea vegetables

**RESISTANT STARCHES
(can be eaten every day in
limited quantities, but those
with prediabetes or diabetes
should use only once or twice
a week on average)**

tortillas (Siete brand—only those
made with cassava and coconut
flour or almond flour)

Siete brand chips (be careful
here, a couple of my canaries
react to the small amount of chia
seeds in the chips)

bread and bagels made by Barely
Bread

Julian Bakery Paleo Wraps (made
with coconut flour) and Paleo
Coconut Flakes Cereal

IN MODERATION

green plantains

green bananas

baobab fruit

cassava (tapioca)

sweet potatoes or yams

rutabaga

parsnips

yucca

celery root (celeriac)

glucomannan (konjac root)

persimmon

jicama

taro root

turnips

tiger nuts

green mango

millet

sorghum

green papaya

**PASTURED POULTRY
(4 ounces per day)**

chicken

turkey

ostrich

pastured or omega-3 eggs (up to
4 daily) Hint: make a four-yolk,
one-white omelet

duck

goose

pheasant

grouse

dove

quail

**MEAT
(100 percent grass-fed,
4 ounces per day)**

bison

wild game

venison

boar

elk

pork (humanely raised)

lamb

beef

prosciutto

PLANT-BASED "MEATS"

Quorn: Chik'n Tenders, Ground,
Chik'n Cutlets, Turk'y Roast,
Bacon-Style Slices

hemp tofu

Hilary's Root Veggie Burger
(hilaryseatwell.com)

tempeh (grain-free only)

The "No, Thank You" List of Lectin-Containing Foods

REFINED, STARCHY FOODS

pasta

rice

potatoes

potato chips

bread

tortillas

pastry

flour

crackers

cookies

cereal

SUGAR

agave

Sweet One of Sunett (acesulfame K)

Splenda (sucralose)

NutraSweet (aspartame)

Sweet'n Low (saccharin)

diet drinks

maltodextrin

VEGETABLES

peas

sugar snap peas

legumes*

green beans

chickpeas* (including as hummus)

soy

tofu

edamame

soy protein

textured vegetable protein (TVP)

pea protein

all beans*, including sprouts

all lentils*

NUTS AND SEEDS

pumpkin

sunflower

chia

peanuts

cashews

**FRUITS
(some called vegetables)**

cucumbers

zucchini

pumpkins

squashes (any kind)

melons (any kind)

eggplant

tomatoes

bell peppers

chili peppers

goji berries

**NON–SOUTHERN EUROPEAN
COW'S MILK PRODUCTS
(these contain casein A1)**

milk

yogurt (including Greek yogurt)

kefir

ice cream

frozen yogurt

cheese

ricotta

cottage cheese

butter, unless from A2 cows, sheep, or goats

**GRAINS, SPROUTED GRAINS,
PSEUDO-GRAINS, & GRASSES**

wheat (pressure-cooking does not remove lectins from any form of wheat)

einkorn wheat

kamut

oats (cannot pressure-cook)

quinoa

rye (cannot pressure-cook)

bulgur

white rice

brown rice

wild rice

barley (cannot pressure-cook)

buckwheat

kasha

spelt

corn

corn products

cornstarch

corn syrup

popcorn

wheatgrass

barley grass

OILS

soy

grape-seed

corn

peanut

cottonseed

safflower

sunflower

"partially hydrogenated"

vegetable

canola

allowable for vegans and vegetarians in phase 2, but only if they are properly prepared in a pressure cooker.

"Maybe" Foods—Foods Whose Lectin Count Can Be Reduced with Preparation

There are some foods on the "no" list that can be made relatively okay in terms of lectins—if you prepare them properly. While I don't advocate eating any of these foods on a regular basis, you can include them in your diet occasionally as long as they don't seem to cause you problems (digestive upset, achiness, brain fog, rashes, et cetera).

BEANS AND LENTILS

For my vegan and vegetarian readers, especially, I know how important beans can be in terms of a go-to, fiber-packed, protein-rich food. However, they are loaded with lectins. In fact, beans are some of the highest-lectin foods there are. The good news is that cooking them in a pressure cooker all but eradicates the lectins in beans and other legumes (as well as many whole grains, but I'll get to that in just a moment). Once those pesky lectins are out of the way, beans become the "healthy" food they're often billed as, because your gut buddies love to feast on their fiber.

So if you want to eat beans often, I recommend investing in an Instant Pot or other pressure cooker (modern iterations of this cooking tool are a far cry from the early versions, which had an unfortunate habit of occasionally exploding). Yet another bonus of pressure-cooking is that it produces perfectly cooked beans in a fraction of the time it takes to cook them on the stove.

If you buy canned beans, I highly suggest you purchase the Eden Foods brand. They pressure-cook their beans right in the cans (which are BPA-free).

Fermentation is another preparation method that dramatically reduces lectin count. If you want to experiment with this age-old technique, fermenting lentils has been shown to reduce their lectin content by 98 percent.[23]

WHEAT AND RICE

Wheat germ agglutinin (WGA) is found in wheat bran, meaning that whole wheat bread has it, but white bread doesn't. And WGA is a dastardly lectin—a much smaller protein than other lectins, WGA can sneak through the gut wall even if your gut barrier is fairly healthy. Once freed from your digestive tract and in your bloodstream, WGA can wreak all kind of havoc—including triggering fat storage, causing neurological problems, and contributing to atherosclerosis. The positive spin on WGA is that it means that delicious, fluffy white bread, naturally raised with yeast or sourdough starters, is actually better for you than the whole wheat/whole grain stuff we think of as "healthy"! By the same token, the bran on rice that makes it brown contains lectins, meaning white rice is actually better for you than the brown rice you've been told is a wiser choice. While I don't recommend eating wheat or rice, per se, if you're going to eat it, eating the de-hulled versions will reduce your lectin exposure. So let's hear it for white bread and white rice! If you're going to eat white bread, to make it even more friendly to your gut wall (and lower in lectins), opt for sourdough, as fermentation also helps reduce lectin content. But let me be very clear: if you have an autoimmune disease or suspect you have one or have a family history, there is no safe wheat bread! And please, pressure-cook your white rice.

There's no point in trying to pressure-cook wheat in an effort to make it more digestible: one lectin that pressure-cooking doesn't remove is gluten. For that reason, there's also no health benefit to pressure-cooking rye, barley, or oats (the other gluten-containing whole grains; even gluten-free oats contain a gluten look-alike lectin).

TOMATOES, PEPPERS, EGGPLANTS, CUCUMBERS, ZUCCHINI

Yes, all of these foods are nightshades, which fall under "just say no" on my list. *But.* I know how much people love these foods. Fresh tomatoes are scrumptious and I realize that folks who live in colder climates look forward to tomato season all year long. To make them more digestible, try to stick to heirloom varieties (which have been around longer than most standard varieties, and thus our microflora and digestive tracts have had at least a smidge more time to acclimate to them) and peel and seed them before you eat them. The best way to peel a tomato is to cut a shallow X on the bottom of them, then drop them in boiling water for a few seconds to loosen the skin. Take them out of the water, let them cool, and then the skin will come right off. Then quarter the tomato and scoop the seeds right out. The blanching doesn't affect the taste.

The same goes for peppers of all kinds—peeling and seeding makes them infinitely more digestible. It's easy enough to seed them; to peel them, I like to briefly roast them either on the grill or directly on the burner of my stove until the skin blisters, making it easy to peel off after putting them in a paper bag for a few minutes to steam.

When it comes to cucumbers, zucchini, and eggplants—if you choose to eat these foods, peel them and seed them if possible. "Baby" versions of these foods are often easier to work with because they contain fewer seeds. When shopping for eggplants, look for those that have a round bottom as opposed to an oval bottom—they are thought to contain fewer seeds.[24]

Fun fact: Americans and Europeans actively shunned tomatoes up until the mid-1800s when Colonel Robert Johnson publicly ate a basket of tomatoes on the Salem, New Jersey, courthouse steps to prove that he wouldn't die or go insane (neither of which happened), so feared were these deadly nightshades.

"Health" Foods That Aren't Actually Healthy

I know how frustrating it is to try to stay on top of which foods are currently considered "healthy" and which aren't, as the guidelines always seem to be changing. I suspect, though, that you will be relieved to see that many of the foods you've been encouraged to eat because they are allegedly "healthy" aren't actually doing you any favors.

Below is a list of so-called "health" foods that really aren't so healthy, as well as the healthier (and oftentimes tastier, in my opinion) alternatives.

"HEALTH" FOOD	BETTER ALTERNATIVE	"HEALTH" FOOD	BETTER ALTERNATIVE
WHOLE WHEAT BREAD	white bread or, even better, sourdough white bread	brown rice	white rice
TOFU	tempeh	beans and lentils	pressure-cooked beans and lentils
PEANUT BUTTER	almond butter	canola, sunflower, or safflower oils	olive oil, coconut oil, or avocado oil
PEANUTS AND CASHEWS	walnuts, pistachios, macadamias	milk and cow's milk cheese	goat's milk, goat cheese and cheeses made from sheep's milk
FREE-RANGE POULTRY AND EGGS	pastured poultry and eggs	raw peppers	roasted, peeled, and seeded peppers
YOGURT	coconut yogurt or goat's milk yogurt (unsweetened)	quinoa	millet

The Truth About Animal Protein

As you probably know, protein is an important macronutrient; your body needs protein to create energy and to maintain muscle. The amino acids in protein are the building blocks of the cells and tissues in the human body—they are literally the stuff we're made of. But here's the thing about protein: you need a lot less of it of it than you probably think you need. And if you're currently eating a typical American diet, or adhering to a Paleo, Whole30, or low-carb eating plan, chances are you're eating *way* too much of it.

I know what you might be thinking—if protein is so essential, how is it possible to eat too much of it? Well, any protein that your body doesn't need right away gets converted into glucose by the liver. Glucose gets stored as fat. It also raises blood sugar levels and insulin levels, and that can lead to a whole host of chronic diseases. On top of that, some of the amino acids in meat appear to be growth agents for cancer and accelerators of aging.[25]

To meet your body's needs, you only need *0.37 grams of protein per kilogram of body weight.*[26] A kilogram equals 2.2 pounds. So, if you weigh 150 pounds, you only need about 25 grams of protein each day. If you weigh 125 pounds, it's 21 grams. To find your target protein allotment, divide your weight by 2.2 to see how much you weigh in kilograms. Then multiply that number by .37 and you've got your answer.

To give you an idea of what 20 grams of protein looks like on your plate, it translates to roughly three ounces of animal protein—about the size of a deck of cards—one Quest bar, or two and a half eggs. When it comes to animal protein, I want you to keep this phrase in mind: "One and you're done." You really don't need to have it at every meal. Have one full portion a day, or spread it throughout the day—say, one egg in the morning, a scoop of goat cheese on your salad at lunch, and a few pieces of shrimp at dinner.

Plants contain less protein than animals, but if you're eating a mostly plant-based diet, it adds up pretty quickly. Half a cup of steamed cauliflower contains one gram of protein, a medium baked sweet potato provides about two grams, and an artichoke has about four grams.

Intermittent Fasting

I love to talk about what to eat—and what to avoid eating—in order to promote your health. But there's another diet strategy that's also important: not eating anything. Or, in other words, fasting. Let's go back to thinking about evolution: our ancestors fasted regularly. Not because it was trendy, but because food simply wasn't always available. Your body is designed to not only withstand periods without food, but to thrive because of them. Over thousands of years, our bodies adapted to be able to process and store energy based on intermittent periods of having access to food and not having access to food. Nowadays, we've got access out the wazoo, and it's contributing to our obesity epidemic and high rates of chronic disease.

Going without food from time to time gives your body a chance to process and digest. It also naturally guides you to reduce your overall caloric intake. And there are many ways to do it.

SOME OPTIONS INCLUDE:

- Choosing two days a week to consume only 500–600 calories—many of my patients find that doing so on Mondays and Thursdays is pretty convenient and easy to do. Mondays, after all, you're naturally ready to cut back after the laxness of the weekend, and Thursday you've had two days of eating normally behind you and the weekend to look forward to. My patients who follow this method tend to lose about a pound a week.

- Try going sixteen hours between your last meal on the day before and your first meal of the next day. So, if you finish eating dinner at 6:00 p.m., don't eat breakfast the next day until 10:00 a.m. Or, if you finish dinner at 8:00 p.m., don't eat until noon the next day.

- Adopt a seasonal intermittent fasting schedule. For example, from January to May of each year, I only eat between 6:00 p.m. and 8:00 p.m. each day. Up until dinner, I drink plenty of green tea and mint tea, and have a cup of coffee each morning. I've been doing this for ten years, so I know it's not only possible, it's sustainable.

Sample Breakfasts, Lunches, and Dinners

I am throwing a lot of nutritional information at you in this chapter, and while the lists of "yes, please" and "no, thank you" foods make things pretty clear, sometimes it's helpful to think about what a typical day of eating might look like. So let's pause for a moment to imagine a typical day on the Plant Paradox plan.

Let's say it's a busy weekday; you've got work and an event afterward. For breakfast, you can scramble two eggs in an ample amount of olive oil. If you want something even quicker, you can grab a coconut-milk, goat-milk, or sheep-milk yogurt and toss in a handful of chopped walnuts or pecans. Or maybe you'll decide to intermittently fast and not eat until mid-late morning. For a snack, you can munch on some plantain chips, or eat half an avocado sprinkled with sea salt (you can even eat it straight out of the peel with a spoon). For lunch you can pack a thermos of leftover Dr. G's Bean Chili (page 129) or Pressure Cooker Black Bean Soup with Avocado Salsa (page 138). And for a fast dinner you can use frozen cauliflower rice to make Cauliflower-Ginger Fried Rice (page 185) and top it off with a couple Dried Fig "Truffles" (page 229). Not bad for a minimal amount of cooking, right?

On a weekend, when you've got a bit more time, you can make yourself a Spanish-ish Omelet (page 115), or really go to town and whip up some Coconut Macadamia Waffles (page 103). For lunch you might have a Banh Mi Bowl (page 146), and then for dinner make a hearty Root Vegetable Lasagna (page 182) or Spinach Artichoke Lasagna (page 181).

There are also plenty of fast, everyday type recipes in this cookbook—Dr. G's Plant-Powered Coffee (page 246) that my wife and I start most days with, for example, or my Dr. Gundry's Nut Mix 2.0 (page 79) that provides a grab-and-go snack that is delicious and filling and that so many of my patients and readers report loving.

While I recognize that you may look at the "no, thank you" list and think that you will never be able to find enough foods to eat to keep your belly full and palate satisfied, I promise you, having a few boundaries is ultimately liberating. When you narrow your choices, it's actually easier to decide what to eat. And once you start experiencing the benefits of eating fewer lectins—less indigestion and bloating, more weight loss, more energy, and fewer aches and pains—you will not feel like you're making any kind of sacrifice.

chapter three

The Plant Paradox Program

By this point in the book, you're probably tired of the word "lectin." You get it. You've read through lists of foods to eat and foods to avoid.

The only piece of the puzzle left is putting together a structured eating plan that makes losing weight and healing your gut effortless.

That's where the Plant Paradox program comes in. This three-phase eating plan provides guidelines for what, how, and when to eat for either the next several weeks or, if you become a convert to this lifestyle like so many of my patients, the rest of your life. The plan is designed to give your body a vacation from the foods that are harming it and provide space for your exquisitely designed healing mechanisms to kick in.

But I do want to be clear that you don't need to follow this program to the letter. If you aren't experiencing any health issues, by all means, skip this chapter and head straight to the recipes. I'm including the program here only so that if, for example, you've loaned out your copy of *The Plant Paradox* to a friend (and they never returned it!), you have everything you need to take the information I covered at length in that book and run with it. My goal is to empower you with information and choices. To that end, here are the guidelines of the Plant Paradox program.

The Four Rules

RULE #1 What You Remove from Your Diet Has a Far Bigger Impact on Your Health Than What You Add to It

Most mainstream diet advice you'll find—in a magazine article, say, or a blog post—will use up a lot of words describing the miraculous health benefits of a particular food or a specific nutrient that is found in a variety of foods. "Munch on macadamia nuts!" "Prioritize antioxidants!" "Eat more omega-3s!" While these individual foods or nutrients may indeed be health-promoting, eating a handful of them on top of a crappy diet isn't going to work miracles. The benefit of any nutritious food is severely limited if the bulk of your diet is sabotaging your health.

I intentionally listed this rule first, because if you do nothing more than remove from your diet the high-lectin foods on the "no" list, I practically guarantee that your health will improve dramatically. Your gut health is so important to every other facet of your well-being, it's no wonder that Hippocrates stated "all disease begins in the gut." Remove the foods that attack your gut wall and wipe out your gut buddies, and your health will flourish.

RULE #2   Take Care of Your Gut Buddies, and They Will Take Care of You

The typical American has been waging an all-out war on his or her microbiome. Antibiotics, antacids, ibuprofen and other nonsteroidal anti-inflammatory drugs, pesticide-laden foods, and a high-sugar, low-fiber diet all decimate your friendly microbes. When you stop eating the foods that wipe out your gut buddies, they will thrive and grow in numbers. When that happens, they crowd out the harmful bacteria and other "gang members" that have been running the show and making you sick. To take it one step further, when you start eating the foods that feed your gut buddies (like many of those on the "yes, please" list in Chapter 2) it's like you become the superhero version of yourself—you become mentally sharper and more impervious to disease. To quote Bette Midler, your gut buddies become the wind beneath your wings.

When you give the bacteria the nutrients they need to thrive, they in turn signal to your immune system that everything is cool—no need for an inflammatory response. And the immune system isn't the only system your gut buddies are talking to—these bacteria communicate with your brain and with all your mitochondria, which are energy-producing organelles located in every cell of your body. Remember, your body is literally a condominium for trillions of bugs, and the more you take care of your tenants, the more your tenants will take care of you.

RULE #3   Fruit Might as Well Be Candy

I know this idea is uncomfortable to accept; it runs counter to everything you've ever been told about fruit. But I implore you to reconsider fruit as "health food." Does fruit contain nutrients? Yes. It contains some fiber, which feeds your gut buddies and promotes your digestion and elimination, and polyphenols, which are naturally-occurring compounds with antioxidant properties. Can you find those nutrients in other food sources? For the most part, yes. There are some polyphenols, such as resveratrol, that are found only in specific fruits (in the case of resveratrol, it's most plentiful in the skin of red grapes), but there are also plenty of polyphenols in greens and cruciferous vegetables.

Let's consider what else fruit contains: lectins and sugar. The peels and seeds of many fruits are typically loaded with lectins, particularly if they have been picked before fully ripening. Remember, fruit isn't just what you typically think of—apples, oranges, berries, bananas, et cetera—it's anything that contains seeds, including tomatoes, cucumbers, and eggplants (all of which are a double whammy: nightshades *and* fruits). And the sugar content of fruit is troublesome. In addition to cueing your body to store fat for the winter, the sugar in fruit is fructose, and fructose is the preferred form of fuel for cancer cells.[27] All sugar, including the sugar in fruit, also causes an immediate spike in blood sugar and insulin, which triggers an inflammatory response from your immune system. I think of eating a bowl of fruit for breakfast as the nutritional equivalent of eating a bowl of Skittles—that's how much I believe the health benefits of fruit have been overrated.

If you're a fruit lover, it's not all bad news. Remember, there are several fruits that are fine to eat: bananas, papayas, and mangoes are a part of the plan, as long as you consume them when they are unripe (green). These unripe fruits are a great source of resistant starches, and resistant starches are a feast for your gut buddies. You may cringe at the thought of eating a green banana, but green banana flour is a great grain substitute in pancakes and baked goods. And sliced green mango and papaya are great additions to salads. (You may also recognize green papaya salad from Thai and Vietnamese restaurant menus—it is tangy and so refreshing!) There are also some fruits on the "yes, please" list of foods that are okay to eat in small amounts when they are in season. Finally, the pulp of fruit and the skin of ripe fruit have the most benefits: get out your juicer, juice your favorite fruits, throw out the juice (yes, pour it down the drain), and eat the pulp and skin that is in the discard bucket! Freeze it in ice cube trays and add a cube or two to your next smoothie.

And there is one fruit you can eat in its ripe stage as much as you please: our dear friend the avocado. With nary a trace of sugar and plenty of good fat and soluble fiber, it's the best fruit you can eat!

RULE #4 You Are What the Thing You Are Eating Ate

This is an important consideration that so many otherwise health-minded folks let slip by. You might choose your produce carefully and go grain-free, but if you're eating animal protein that is anything other than pasture-raised, you're not eating as cleanly as you think you are. Cows, pigs, and chickens that are fattened up on corn or soy or wheat ingest a lot of lectins in those foods; you consume these lectins (along with other stuff, like antibiotics) when you consume the animal. If you remove high-lectin foods from your diet but still eat conventionally raised animal protein or farmed fish or seafood, you're sabotaging yourself. Honestly, this was a hard one for even me to believe at first, but for so many of my patients, the final obstacle standing in their way to great health was this one simple rule.

———————

These are the broad strokes of the Plant Paradox program, and if you want to refine your efforts beyond simply removing the foods on the "No" list, these are the principles that will help guide you back to a level of vitality you likely haven't felt in years. The three-phase plan that follows is meant to be implemented from start to finish—you begin at Phase 1, cycle through Phase 2, and complete Phase 3, or perhaps stay on Phase 3 forever. That said, if you're in relatively good health already and aren't looking to lose weight, you can skip the Phase 1 cleanse if you'd like.

PHASE #1 A Three-Day Kick-Start Cleanse

Imagine, if you will, your gut as an empty lot—a weed-infested, totally overgrown, vines-choking-out-every-tree kind of empty lot—with a fence surrounding it that is riddled with holes, so all manner of varmints have taken up residence in the scraggly environs. Got the picture?

In order to transform this eyesore into a vibrant, beautiful, and thriving ecosystem, the first thing you've got to do is get rid of the weeds. In my experience treating tens of thousands of patients, I have seen proof again and again that if your gut is a breeding ground for unfriendly bacteria, yeast, fungi, and other gang members, it doesn't matter how many healthy foods you eat; your body simply won't be able to process them any more than organic seeds planted in a completely overgrown field will sprout, grow, and thrive. You've got to make space for health to set in—and mend those holes in the fence of your gut garden—by clearing out the invasive species that have taken over. And according to many well-designed studies,[28,29,30] your microbiome responds quickly to a change in diet, meaning that a short-term dietary shake-up (like Phase 1) is an effective way to immediately change the makeup of your gut's bacterial population.

From here, because you won't want those icky bad guys to reassert themselves, you'll want to move right into Phase 2. Meaning, if you think you can do a three-day cleanse and then go back to your old eating habits, and still experience lasting benefits to your health, you're wrong. (Bummer, I know.) I call Phase 1 a kick-start because it lays the foundation for the eating strategies you'll employ in Phase 2 to show their benefits more quickly. But Phase 1 is optional. If you choose to jump right into Phase 2, just be patient, as it will probably take a bit longer for you to notice results.

There are three parts to Phase 1:

PART 1: Do not eat *any* dairy, grains (including pseudo-grains such as quinoa), fruit, sugar, seeds, eggs, soy, nightshades, roots, or tubers. No corn, soy, or canola oils, or any form of beef or conventionally-raised meats. Removing these foods will help quell inflammation and starve your unfriendly microbes. Basically, you eat nothing but organic vegetables from the "yes, please" list, as well as avocado and small amounts of wild-caught fish, pastured chicken, tempeh, shellfish, hemp tofu, or certain Quorn products (listed on the "yes, please" list), and healthy fats and approved nuts.

Just for Phase 1 and the first two weeks of Phase 2, also avoid extra-virgin olive oil and coconut oil because they allow lipopolysaccharides (LPS), a bacterial cell wall component that closely resembles the chemical structure of lectins, to hitch a ride through the gut wall where they then trigger an immune response—and you don't want to give your body any extra work to do during this time. Instead, use macadamia nut oil, walnut oil, avocado oil, ghee, MCT oil, or perilla oil (a popular cooking oil in Asia that's available in Asian markets, at Whole Foods, and from online sources). You can drink all the water and black and green tea (sweetened only with stevia) you'd like. Appropriate recipes for this phase include Garlic-and-Walnut-Stuffed Mushrooms (page 92), Ralph's Breakfast Scramble (the vegan version, page 99), Lemon, Kale, and Chicken Soup (page 133), and Tangy Coconut Greens (page 212).

PART 2: Optionally, you can assist in your body's efforts to get rid of any "weeds" in your gut by taking a gentle laxative. I recommend an herbal blend called Swiss Kriss, which has an active ingredient of senna. It is available at most pharmacies and online. Take two tablets at bedtime along with a glass of water the night before you start Phase 1 (you only need to do this on the first day, no need to repeat on days 2 and 3). Oh, by the way, it helps to be home the next morning, as Swiss Kriss tends to work quickly.

PART 3: If you suffer from digestive disorders such as IBS, leaky gut, or any autoimmune condition, consider taking supplements that aid in killing unfriendly gut bugs, including: berberine (found in Oregon grape root extract), grapefruit seed extract (*not* grape-seed extract), and mushroom extracts. I provide specific dosage information in the Resources section at the back of the book (page 267). Spices that help support digestive healing include black pepper, cloves, cinnamon, and wormwood, so be sure to use these in your cooking or consume them as a supplement.

You may feel hungry, cranky, or tired during these seventy-two hours. I will probably not be your favorite person during this time! But at the end of your three days, you should have lost a few pounds (up to 4 is typical) and reduced your inflammation to the point that you notice you don't feel as achy. Your balance of gut bacteria should also be tilted much more toward the friendly guys outnumbering the unfriendly ones.

Remember, despite starting to feel better, reverting back to your old food habits will only tip the scale back in favor of the unfriendly bacterial and fungal domination, so on the morning of Day 4, head straight into Phase 2.

PHASE #2 Repair and Restore for Six Weeks

In this phase of the program, you are basically retraining your eating habits so that you create a healthy digestive environment that continues to nurture your gut buddies and doesn't let the bad guys come roaring back and take over the place. If Phase 1 was about pulling the weeds in the overgrown garden of your digestive tract, Phase 2 is about nurturing the soil and rebuilding the fences that keep unwelcome critters out of your crops. In my experience, it takes people six weeks to fully establish a new habitual eating pattern; for that reason, Phase 2 of the Plant Paradox program lasts for six weeks.

I know how hard it is to break old patterns and addictive behaviors. What is likely to happen on this phase of the plan is that a couple weeks in, you will start to feel great. Your clothes will be looser, your energy will soar, and you may be tempted to start thinking, "I'm now so healthy that I can go back to eating whatever I want." Please, I beg you—stick with this part of the program for a full six weeks. Even though the benefits that you'll start feeling are real, it takes time to seal up those holes in your gut wall; the bad guys are looking for any opportunity to regain the upper hand. You've got to show them no mercy and starve them out—it's the best way to give yourself the healing you need and deserve.

In this phase of the plan, you'll continue to avoid everything on the "no, thank you" list (page 32), steer clear of all fruit except for those allowed on Phase 1, avoid cow's milk dairy as much as possible (although coconut milk and yogurt are okay; as are milk, cheese, and yogurt made from sheep and goat milk so long as you don't overdo them because they do contain Neu5Gc), and omit beans and tofu and other unfermented soy products (for everyone, but this is of particular note if you are a vegetarian or a vegan—I'll give some specific guidance for my non-meat-eating friends at the end of this chapter). As with Phase 1, for the first two weeks of Phase 2, limit your consumption of coconut oil and olive oil. Since we're trying to cool inflammation as much as possible during this early phase of the program, easing off these oils will help you meet that goal, at least for now. After two weeks on Phase 2, you can begin to add these oils back into your normal rotation.

You are free to consume up to eight ounces of animal protein a day (only from pastured animals, omega-3 eggs, or wild-caught seafood, preferably in two four-ounce portions a day—about the size of the palm of your hand), but I would prefer that you eat less of these proteins. You should also maximize your resistant starch intake to fuel your rehabbed gut buddies—plantains, sweet potatoes or yams, taro root, shirataki noodles (a tasty pasta alternative found in the grocery store refrigerator case), parsnips, turnips, jicama, celery root, Jerusalem artichokes (also known as sunchokes), as well as green mangoes, papayas, and bananas. Other foods that help feed your friendly bacteria are radicchio, Belgian endive, okra, artichokes, onions, garlic, and mushrooms—they provide an indigestible (to humans) sugar called inulin that good bacteria love.

Your gut buddies also love leafy greens and cruciferous vegetables, so continue to eat plenty of these (as you did in Phase 1). Like I mentioned in Rule 4, another surprising way to feed your gut buddies the polyphenols they love without also delivering a healthy dose of sugars that the bad bacteria love is to get out your fruit juicer and use it in reverse—throw the juice away and eat the pulp that's left behind. You can add it to a smoothie, stir it into some coconut, goat, or sheep yogurt, or mix it into your salad dressing. Nuts are a great snack for this phase, particularly polyphenol-rich pistachios, walnuts, macadamias, and pecans, up to a half cup a day. Fresh or dried figs (which are technically a flower and not a fruit) and dates are good sources of the fibers only your good gut buddies love, and are great to use in limited amounts when you need a sweet boost—add them to salads or smoothies.

Some of the recipes that you can enjoy in Phase 2 include Cheesy Cauliflower Muffins (page 101), Chocolate Chip Mini-Pancakes (page 104), Beef and Mushroom Stew (page 140), Shrimp Poke Bowl (page 149), and Creamy Shrimp and Kale Spaghetti (page 156).

In addition, in Phase 2 you'll start taking a fish oil capsule—one that contains the highest number of milligrams of DHA that you can afford. Ideally you'll consume a total 1,000 mg of DHA a day—either before each meal or by mixing flavored cod liver oil with a healthy oil from the "yes, please" list. If you're a vegan or vegetarian, take an algal DHA capsule instead. The other vital supplement to add to your daily regimen is Vitamin D_3. Aim for taking 5,000 to 10,000 IUs a day, unless you are working with a health-care provider who is monitoring your levels and counseling you to take more. In my fifteen years of practicing restorative medicine, I have regularly prescribed up to an astonishing 40,000 IUs a day to get vitamin D levels up to at least 70 ng/ml, which is what I consider to be the floor of a healthy baseline (I keep my levels, and those of my autoimmune and cancer patients, greater than 100 ng/ml).

The final piece of the puzzle here is to stop taking—if possible, and with the guidance of your health-care provider, of course—any prescription drugs that disrupt your microbiome, including antibiotics, stomach-acid-blocking drugs (replace with Rolaids, Tums, DGL, or marshmallow root), and NSAIDS (such as ibuprofen and naproxen; replace with Tylenol or boswellia extract).

PHASE #3 Reap the Rewards

When my patients come to see me after they've been on the Plant Paradox program for at least six weeks (whether or not they jump-started with a Phase 1 cleanse), I see and hear all kinds of amazing things. They've lost excess weight or gained a few pounds if they were underweight. If they've been suffering from arthritis or an autoimmune condition, they marvel at how much their chronic pain has dissipated. Their digestion is improved and any constipation or diarrhea has rectified itself. They also understand that they haven't merely completed a diet; they have changed their bodies for the better—and they want to keep feeling good.

In this final phase of the Plant Paradox program, you can start to reintroduce certain lectin-containing foods—with proper preparation. Doing so not only expands your food choices, it gives you a chance to fully understand just how much your gut has healed and your gut buddies have resumed control of your intestines and your immune system. You don't have to make this shift exactly at the six-week mark—if you are feeling great and don't want to modify your eating plan, by all means, keep going until you feel some natural desire to change things up.

If any of the following conditions *haven't* been met, I encourage you to keep going with Phase 2 until they are resolved:

- Bowel movements have become regular
- Joints have stopped hurting
- Brain fog has receded
- Skin has cleared
- Energy has risen noticeably
- Sleep has improved
- Weight has normalized

Some of you are simply more sensitive to lectins than others. If you are hypothyroid, have arthritis or heart disease, have a diagnosed autoimmune disease, have had your tonsils or appendix removed, or have chronic sinus issues, I advise you to stick to Phase 2; you wouldn't want to neutralize the health benefits you've just spent six weeks cultivating with one serving of beans, would you?

The majority of you reading this, however, are not canaries. So when you feel ready to start reintroducing some foods, consider yourself on Phase 3 of the Plant Paradox program. Honestly, this phase can last a lifetime, as it is more of a lifestyle than a diet.

Continuing with the foods you ate and strategies you implemented in

Phase 2, at this point you can start eating more coconut oil, introducing "baby" versions of lectin-containing foods such as cucumbers, zucchini, and Japanese eggplant (because these immature versions contain few or no seeds), as well as peeled and seeded heirloom tomatoes and peppers. Next comes pressure-cooked beans and lentils in small amounts. If you tolerate those well, then try small servings of pressure-cooked white basmati rice (preferably from India) or pressure cooked pseudo-grains like quinoa. In terms of timing, reintroduce no more than one new food a week so that you can assess the effect each has on you and your microbiome. If you can pinpoint one or two troublesome foods by watching your bowel movements, your joints, your skin, and your mood, you can take extra care to avoid them while enjoying some of the other new foods that don't cause a negative reaction.

In general, you want to continue to reduce your consumption of beef, pork, or lamb (even though it's pastured or wild) because of its Neu5Gc content; I suggest working toward a maximum of two ounces a day. Then start reducing the other safer animal proteins like fish and chicken. Remember, nuts, leaves, and mushrooms all have plenty of protein to meet your body's needs. Every time you worry about getting enough protein from leaves, check out the muscles on a gorilla or a horse!

You also want to keep your fruit intake to a very moderate amount, and limit it to either unripe fruit or fruit that is in season, and then remove the peels and seeds of the fruit you do consume. I also recommend you limit your intake of acceptable dairy from goat, sheep, and Southern European cows (see the "yes, please" list), because they also contain Neu5Gc. And as much as your gut buddies love the resistant starches in tubers, if you over-rely on these foods they will lead to weight gain, so keep your plate filled mostly with vegetables and limit resistant starches to a supporting role—not the star of the show. You also want to develop your habits around going longer between meals and implementing intermittent fasting (turn to page 37 for more information on this). Stick with the supplement routine I outlined for Phase 2, and to really send your health soaring, make a point of exposing yourself to more natural sunlight—an hour a day is the goal. Try for eight hours of sleep each night and get regular exercise. Block out blue light (from phones, computers, televisions, et cetera) at night and avoid the endocrine disruptors we discussed on page 10.

Foods for Each Phase of the Plant Paradox Program

To make it as simple as possible to know when to eat which foods, I've compiled this at-a-glance list of acceptable foods for each phase of the Plant Paradox program.

PHASE 1

leafy green vegetables—endive, lettuce, spinach, Swiss chard, and watercress

cruciferous vegetables—bok choy, broccoli, Brussels sprouts, cabbage, cauliflower, kale, and mustard greens

artichokes

asparagus

celery

fennel

radishes

fresh herbs including mint, parsley, basil, and cilantro

garlic, onions, leeks, and chives

kelp, seaweed, and nori

wild-caught seafood or pastured poultry, no more than a total of eight ounces a day

Quorn products (see list of "yes, please" foods for acceptable options)

tempeh (grain-free version)

hemp tofu

avocado, up to one a day

olives

avocado oil, macadamia nut oil, walnut oil, hemp seed oil, flaxseed oil, MCT oil, perilla oil, ghee

nuts (see "yes, please" food list for specific types)

lemon juice

vinegar

mustard

green, black, or herbal tea

coffee

stevia or Just Like Sugar

PHASE 2

All of the foods listed for Phase 1, plus:

moderate amounts of in-season fruit or green bananas, mangoes, or papayas

pastured or omega-3 eggs

plantains

shirataki noodles (sold under the brand name Miracle Noodles)

parsnips

turnips

jicama

celery root

Jerusalem artichokes (sunchokes)

sweet potatoes

almond flour

cassava flour

coconut flour

sorghum

millet

inulin and yacón syrup

okra

radicchio

mushrooms, raw or cooked

plain goat, sheep, or coconut yogurt

figs

dates

extra-virgin olive oil and coconut oil, after two weeks on Phase 2

PHASE 3

All the foods on the Phase 1 and Phase 2 lists, plus:

peeled and seeded baby cucumbers, zucchini, and Japanese eggplants, adding them one at a time to your diet and making sure you don't experience any adverse effects before trying another one

peeled and seeded heirloom tomatoes and peppers, testing one at a time to determine how they affect you

pressure-cooked beans and lentils

pressure-cooked Indian white basmati rice

casein A2 dairy—milk and cheese from goats, sheep, water buffalo, and Southern European cows

white sourdough bread (do not eat if you have or have had an autoimmune disease, diabetes, prediabetes, or cancer)—use only as a sponge to get olive oil into your mouth

A Note for Vegetarians and Vegans

I want to be very clear: I am pro-vegetarian and vegan, and so is the Plant Paradox program. After all, I was a professor at the Loma Linda University School of Medicine, which is a Seventh-Day Adventist vegetarian institution, for sixteen years. I have also studied the research into the blue zones—the areas of the world where people live the longest, as portrayed in journalist Dan Buettner's book *The Blue Zones*—and have taken to heart that these diets advocate eating far less animal protein than is standard in the American diet. And yet, here I am, advocating that you don't eat many staples of a vegetarian diet, including rice, beans, tofu, and pasta. What gives?

When you look more closely at the dietary similarities between the inhabitants of the blue zones, you realize that they don't rely on whole grains and beans as much as many people assume. If you look at the diets of Okinawans, for example, 70 percent of their calories come from a purple sweet potato. Six percent of their diet is white rice, another 6 percent is soy (in the forms of tofu and miso), and the rest was a smattering of pork and vegetables. In the Seventh-Day Adventist community in Loma Linda, 50 percent of their calories come from fat, regardless if they are vegetarian or vegan. Their main protein source is TVP (texturized vegetarian protein), a defatted soy protein, which is pressure-cooked and extruded under high pressure and heat. Remember this: the Adventists use pressure-cooked "beans." In Acciaroli, Italy, a newly discovered blue zone, most of their calories come from olive oil, anchovies, and rosemary; they eat minimal meat and grain, and have a higher concentration of people over one hundred than any other place in the world. By the way, they also drink red wine every day and smoke like fiends.

I believe that the main reason why people in the blue zones live longer is because they eat a low percentage of animal protein, and not necessarily the high percentage of grains and beans that pro-bean and -grain proponents claim they eat. You really do want to moderate your meat and animal product consumption (including eggs and cheese)—no matter how well the animals were raised—because all animal protein ages us. As explained previously, animal protein contains a sugar molecule called Neu5Gc, which makes our immune system attack the lining of our blood vessels, contributing to heart disease and cancer. In addition, and this is really bizarre, cancer cells use Neu5Gc to hide from the immune system. It's a cloaking device—when we look at the chemical composition of tumors, we see that they are full of Neu5Gc. Finally, certain amino acids that stimulate the aging receptor mTOR are far more concentrated in animal protein, including chicken and fish, as opposed to plant proteins. So, vegetarians and vegans, I want you to know that I consider you to be very much ahead of the game when it comes to staying as young as possible as you age. But sadly, certain of your protein sources, unless properly prepared, are making you sicker rather than healthier.

I don't want to take away anyone's beloved rice and beans. So long as you respect that these plants never wanted to be eaten—or their babies to be eaten—and take steps to cook them properly (with a pressure cooker, which destroys lectins), you will be okay. I have been so impressed by my patients' stories of how their grandmothers in Brazil or Peru always used a pressure cooker to prepare beans, or rice, or quinoa, and that it was when my patients stopped this "old-fashioned" practice that they became ill. It turns out Grandma knew a thing or two. With the lectins removed, beans offer a delicious feast of soluble fiber and resistant starch for your gut buddies. With just a little bit of knowledge and wise choices, you *can* eat moderate quantities of beans and legumes starting in Phase 2. Rice should probably wait until Phase 3, but it too isn't off the table. The only thing that really should stay off your plate for the long term are wheat, rye, barley, and oats, as pressure-cooking does not destroy their lectin content.

Plant Paradox Program for Life: A New Food Pyramid

Now that you're ready to incorporate the Plant Paradox as a long-term lifestyle, let's talk less about lists and more about what the overall composition of your diet should look like moving forward. To that end, I've created a quick and easy reference for you: the Plant Paradox Food Pyramid.

At first glance, it looks very similar to the standard food pyramid created by the U.S. Department of Agriculture's Center for Nutrition Policy and Promotion, which I've included below my pyramid just to refresh your memory.

It has the same triangular shape and shows you which foods to eat the most of and which foods to eat sparingly. But that is where the similarities

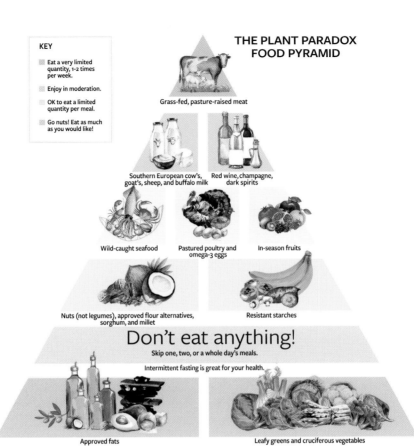

THE PLANT PARADOX FOOD PYRAMID

KEY

- Eat a very limited quantity, 1–2 times per week.
- Enjoy in moderation.
- OK to eat a limited quantity per meal.
- Go nuts! Eat as much as you would like!

Grass-fed, pasture-raised meat

Southern European cow's, goat's, sheep, and buffalo milk

Red wine, champagne, dark spirits

Wild-caught seafood

Pastured poultry and omega-3 eggs

In-season fruits

Nuts (not legumes), approved flour alternatives, sorghum, and millet

Resistant starches

Don't eat anything!

Skip one, two, or a whole day's meals.

Intermittent fasting is great for your health.

Approved fats

Leafy greens and cruciferous vegetables

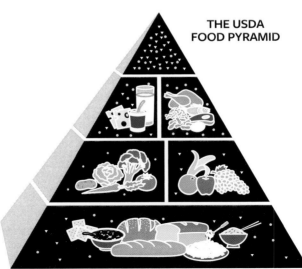

THE USDA FOOD PYRAMID

Source: U.S. Department of Agriculture/U.S. Department of Health and Human Services

end. Whereas the USDA's food pyramid will put on you a fast track to digestive ailments, chemical contamination, and a host of diseases, the Plant Paradox Food Pyramid will help you find and maintain your ideal weight and dramatically reduce the inflammation at the root of so many chronic diseases. If you'd like to print out a copy to hang on your fridge (as opposed to tearing out a page of this beautiful book), visit: gundrymd.com/wp-content/pdf/Gundry_Food_Pyramid.pdf.

What's so wrong with the standard food pyramid? Well, for starters, look at the foundation of it—it suggests you eat primarily grains in the form of bread, pasta, cereal, and more bread. Because these items are so highly processed, this is one of the food groups that is mostly like to contain dastardly food additives and deadly disruptors.

For instance, bread products often contain added preservatives and ingredients like food dyes, high-fructose corn syrup, or even the dangerous chemical azodicarbonamide—aka the yoga-mat chemical. That's the material put in sandals and yoga mats to give them cushion; it was put in bread for years as a bleaching agent or to make the bread fluffy.

Beyond that, the old food pyramid makes it seem like eating eleven slices of bread is not only okay, but health promoting. By the way, Sardinians (one of the Blue Zones) do eat up to eleven slices of bread a day, but they have the highest incidence of autoimmune disease in Europe! And since wheat flour is loaded with lectins such as gluten and wheat germ agglutinin (WGA), it attacks our gut wall and cues the storage of belly fat.

Perhaps the biggest difference between my food pyramid and the standard USDA model is this first, foundational level. As you can see, I don't have grains anywhere near the bottom of the pyramid. Rather, I advise that you make the major components of your diet healthy fats, leafy greens, and cruciferous vegetables. These foods are so supportive of health that you can consume them in unlimited quantities. They include:

- extra-virgin olive oil, avocado oil, walnut oil, sesame oil, and coconut oil

- avocados

- romaine, red and green leaf lettuce, kohlrabi, mesclun (baby greens), spinach, endive, butter lettuce, parsley, fennel, seaweed/sea vegetables

- broccoli, cauliflower, Brussels sprouts, bok choy, cabbage, asparagus, and radishes

The second level of the food pyramid is perhaps the most mind-blowing part—because it doesn't contain any food at all! Rather, I suggest that you find a way to incorporate intermittent fasting into your regular eating schedule, whether that's eating each day only during a compressed window of time (between the hours of 10:00 a.m. and 6:00 p.m., say), or restricting your intake to 500 or so calories for one or two days a week, or whatever strategy works best for you. Because our bodies adapted to regular cycles of feasting and famine as our species evolved, it actually benefits us to go without food from time to time. Intermittent fasting is one of the keys to overall health, and that's the reason it's the second pillar of the pyramid.

The third tier of the Plant Paradox Food Pyramid consists of nuts, flour alternatives, and lectin-free grains. This is where you can satisfy those grain and bread cravings. And yes, it's okay to indulge in this category daily, but make sure to limit consumption of these foods to small portions per meal. With cassava flour, almond flour, tapioca flour, and coconut flour, you can recreate many of your favorite baked goods. And with sorghum and millet, two lectin-free grains, you can make alternatives for favorite dishes like stuffing and tabbouleh that fit the bill. Next, resistant starches make the list because they feed friendly bacteria. It's okay to eat them every day, but limit the quantity with each meal.

You'll notice that we had to get pretty high up the pyramid before we covered any animal protein (although egg yolks are a good source of healthy fats—you can have up to four of them a day, but ideally only one white; you can feed the extra egg whites to your dog or cat if you have one). The fourth tier of the pyramid includes wild-caught seafood, pastured poultry, and eggs. It also contains fruit, which should be regarded as a treat and eaten in moderation. It's okay to eat a small portion of in-season fruit every day. Just consider that, if you live in a cold climate, there will be several months out of the year when no fruit is in season! Be very moderate with your fruit consumption, and your waistline will thank you. The only fruits that are okay to eat year-round are green bananas, mangoes, papayas, and the ever-faithful avocado.

Up near the top of the pyramid is dairy made from Southern European cows, goats, sheep, and buffalo. These types of milk products are allowed because they're the only milks that contain casein A2 protein and not casein A1. Consider these milk products an indulgence and consume them only in moderate quantities.

Also up at the top is grass-fed or pasture-raised meat from cows, pigs, venison, lamb, bison, and wild game. You want to eat only very small amounts of these meats because they contain Neu5Gc.

At the very tipsy top of the pyramid are certain alcoholic beverages and dark chocolate. Up to one ounce of dark chocolate a day—at least 72 percent cacao—is fine. And red wine in moderation can actually help our health. Moderation in this case means a max of four to six ounces per day, only with meals. And as I covered in Chapter 2, champagne and the darker spirits (such as bourbon and rye) have some health benefits to impart as well.

When you let this new pyramid be your guide, you have a simple graphic representation of a paradigm for healthy living.

chapter four

The Plant Paradox Kitchen

Success on any eating plan starts with having a well-stocked kitchen and pantry that makes meal prep easy, quick, and enjoyable.

When it comes to stocking your pantry, I've tried to keep it so that 90 percent of the ingredients I use are items you can find at Costco, Walmart, or a big grocery store. In fact, while I was working on this list, I would often look up a Walmart in a town in the Midwest to make sure that an item was available there. I've found cassava flour and shirataki noodles at Walmart—you may be surprised what's available if you take the time to look. While I do recommend non-GMO and organic versions of foods whenever possible, I know that their added expense can make following the Plant Paradox program difficult for some people, so I urge you to just do your best.

If you can't find an ingredient at a reasonable price locally, I recommend going online and checking out Amazon or Thrive Market—a website that is a cross between Costco and Whole Foods, offering high-quality foods at lower prices for a yearly membership fee.

It may also seem like you have to buy and acclimate your taste buds to a lot of new and different ingredients, but here's a tip for you: If you want to start with a smaller number of new-to-you ingredients, I advocate for almond flour, cassava flour, and coconut flour. With those three basic ingredients you can make a ton of new recipes, and even swap these out for other alternative flours.

Beyond that, I want to introduce you to some of the staples I turn to again and again both for the recipes included here and in my own pantry. These are my favorites, and once you start eating them regularly, I think they will become your favorites too.

Plant Paradox Pantry Staples

Almond butter: I know what a comforting staple peanut butter can be for a lot of people, but since peanuts are one of the highest-lectin foods out there, it definitely doesn't have a place in the Plant Paradox pantry. In fact, it's a food I argue *everyone* should avoid, whether you care about lectins or not. (Butters made out of cashews or sunflower seeds are no better, because those two foods are also high in lectins.) But don't panic, almond butter is every bit as delicious and it's low in lectins. Preferably you'll spring for the organic version made from raw nuts, but if that is prohibitive for your grocery budget, just be sure to avoid any almond butter that contains partially hydrogenated oils (aka trans fats) and sweeteners of any type.

Almond flour: This flour alternative is nothing more than finely ground almonds, preferably skinless or "blanched," as there are lectins in the skins of almonds. Look for a product that uses non-GMO almonds; bonus points if they are organic. Store this versatile flour in the freezer to keep it fresh longer.

Almond milk: This milk alternative has a nice flavor all on its own—avoid sweetened or flavored versions. As with almond butter and flour, non-GMO is better, and organic is best.

Arrowroot flour: Arrowroot is an herb and this flour—also sometimes labeled "arrowroot starch"—is made from its root. It makes a great thickener, so you can use it in sauces where you would normally use cornstarch. I also like to add it to waffle and pancake batter when using alternative flours, as it helps the batter hold together.

Avocado: These rich, creamy beauties are so healthful I advocate eating as much as one whole one a day. The only hitch is that they need to be ripe when you're ready to eat them. In order to ripen an avocado more quickly, put them near your green bananas, and if you're really in a pinch, you can bake an avocado in a 350-degree oven for 10 minutes to soften it up—the flavor won't be perfect but the texture will be right. Once they're ripe, you can put them in the fridge to make them last another day or two at most, or take them out of the skin, puree them, and then freeze in a freezer bag. I prefer Haas avocados, which have a dark green or black skin with a pebbly texture, but Florida avocados are good too.

Avocado mayonnaise: Most mayonnaise is made with low-quality, high-lectin and GMO soybean oil, or other vegetable oils that are also high in lectins such as safflower or canola oil. Mayonnaise made with avocado oil is your best bet, health-wise. Primal Kitchen makes a great avocado mayo that's available through Thrive Market, or Chosen Foods Avocado Mayo is available at Costco.

Avocado oil: With its high smoke point and mild taste, avocado oil is an excellent all-around cooking oil. Costco and most supermarkets carry it.

Baking powder, aluminum-free: Most baking sodas contain sodium aluminum phosphate or sodium aluminum sulfate, but aluminum is no friend to your health! Two aluminum-free brands to look for are Bob's Red Mill and Rumford.

Basmati rice: In Phase 3, it's okay to start eating very moderate amounts of rice; I recommend that you limit it to white basmati rice because it has the lowest lectin content and high levels of resistant starch of any rice. Look for rice from India, not Texas—remember, we want to eat foods that humans have been eating for a long time, and Texas basmati rice is a very recent addition to the food supply, and is an entirely different grain that has less of the resistant starch you want in your rice.

Cassava flour: Cassava flour comes from the root known as manioc, yucca, or yuca, and is full of resistant starch. It is also the key to fluffy gluten-free baked goods. If you can't find it in your local supermarket, Moon Rabbit and Otto's Naturals brands are available on Amazon.

Cauliflower rice: This savory side dish and building block of many of the recipes in this book isn't actually rice at all—it's finely chopped cauliflower. While you can easily make it yourself by pulsing cauliflower florets in a food processor, buying it premade is incredibly convenient and cost effective. Look for it in the freezer section of Whole Foods, Costco, and Trader Joe's, or fresh in many mainstream grocery stores.

Cayenne pepper: If you love a spicy kick, make sure to skip the red chili flakes—which contain the skins and seeds of hot peppers—and stick to cayenne pepper, which is made of ground pepper after it has been peeled and seeded. The same is true for paprika.

Chocolate: When it comes to purchasing chocolate bars, look for at least 72 percent cacao; there are many options available at regular grocery stores as well as at Costco. Look for organic and fair trade chocolate bars whenever you can, and limit your intake to one ounce or less per day. For baking, look for an unsweetened, high-cacao content chocolate, also at least 72 percent cacao. Some products go as high as 99 percent cacao; World Market sells a 99 percent cacao baking chocolate that has a surprisingly sweet taste. Dagoba and Lily's make excellent chocolate chips.

Cocoa powder: Not to be confused with hot chocolate ("cocoa"), which is a pre-sweetened mix that includes some cocoa powder and a lot of sugar, cocoa powder is simply ground cacao beans. Because on its own cocoa powder can be fairly bitter (which is actually a good thing, as the flavor is a direct result of all the polyphenols cacao contains), many cocoa powders contain potassium bromate or potassium carbonate to neutralize the taste—and the health benefits—of the polyphenols. That means you want to skip Dutch process cocoa powder and look for the words "nonalkalized." My favorite cocoa powders are made by Dagoba or Scharffen Berger.

Coconut aminos: A delicious replacement for soy and tamari, coconut aminos consist of only two ingredients—organic coconut tree sap and organic sea salt. That's it. See, soy's a bean. So, soy sauce is a bean sauce. And beans, as you know, are rife with lectins. Not to mention soy sauce contains wheat, and wheat contains gluten—a pretty offending lectin. I say, skip the whole soy sauce section and use coconut aminos instead.

Coconut cream: This is the rich, creamy part of coconut milk. There are two ways to buy it: you can look for a can of coconut cream (I like the Trader Joe's brand), just be sure to avoid brands with BPA-lined cans or added sugar. If you can't find cans of the cream, you can buy coconut milk and store it in the refrigerator overnight. The cream will rise to the top and harden—just scoop it out gently the next day.

Coconut flour: Another great flour alternative, coconut flour helps you make a wide variety of baked goods. It's a bit denser than other flours, meaning it absorbs more liquid than you might expect, so be sure to follow recipes for a while until you get a better sense of how this flour works with other ingredients before you start experimenting. Some of my favorite brands are Bob's Red Mill, Nutiva, and Let's Do.

Coconut milk: This is the milk alternative that's sold either in the refrigerated dairy case in a cardboard carton or the beverage aisle in a Tetra Pak so that it can be stored at room temperature until you're ready to use it. It has a richer consistency than other nondairy milks, meaning it makes a nice creamy replacement. Look for unsweetened and unflavored versions.

Coconut oil: A great cooking oil because of its high smoke point, coconut oil also makes a great addition to baked goods. Look for extra-virgin coconut oil from brands such as Kirkland, Viva Labs, Carrington Farms, and Nature's Way.

Eggs: I love eggs—in fact, I advocate consuming the yolks more strongly than the whites, because they are a great source of healthy fats and nutrients! My favorite omelet is made from four yolks and one egg white (you can feed the excess egg whites to your pet). Just make sure you buy eggs that are either pastured or omega-3 eggs.

Erythritol: This natural sweetener is a sugar alcohol. Your body processes it differently than traditional sugars—it doesn't cause a spike in blood sugar. It's also less likely to cause stomach upset than other sugar alternatives. Best of all, it acts just like sugar when you bake with it, meaning it dissolves easily into batters and tastes great. It's often sold under the brand name Swerve; Wholesome sells a version of it too.

Flaxseed meal: Flaxseeds are a great source of short-chain omega-3s and contain no lectins. The only hitch is, they need to be ground in order for your body to be able to access those omega-3s, and once they are ground, they are very prone to oxidation. So the best way to add them to your diet is to buy them whole and grind them as needed in a coffee or spice grinder. If you prefer to buy them already ground, look for a product that was cold-milled, as heat can oxidize the fats, and then store it in the freezer to keep it fresh longer.

Ghee: Otherwise known as clarified butter, ghee is butter that has had the milk solids (which consist of protein, including the troublesome casein A1) cooked out of it, making it shelf stable and easily digestible. Look for ghee made from the milk of grass-fed cows, which has a higher amount of omega-3s than conventionally raised cows fed a diet of corn and soy. Pure and Pure Indian Foods are two grass-fed brands to look for.

Goat's milk, cheese, and yogurt: Goat's milk also doesn't contain casein A1 (unlike most cow's milk) and so it makes a more gut-friendly alternative to traditional dairy. You can also use goat cheese, sometimes known as chèvre, and goat's milk yogurt or kefir (stick to unsweetened, unflavored varieties).

Hemp milk: Yes, this is the same hemp that is kin to marijuana (although eating or drinking it will not give you a high). This is yet another alternative to cow's milk that's great in smoothies and other recipes. Again, stick to the unsweetened, unflavored varieties.

Hemp protein powder: A great alternative to whey protein powder for vegans or anyone who wants to reduce their intake of animal protein, hemp protein powder provides all the essential amino acids and plenty of omega-3s.

Hemp tofu: Another way to enjoy the nutritional benefits of hemp is with this more densely textured alternative to traditional tofu. You can find the non-GMO Living Harvest Tempt brand of hemp tofu at Whole Foods.

Honey: Although honey is a natural sugar, it is still sugar and should be consumed only in very small amounts—one teaspoon or less a day—only in Phase 3 of the Plant Paradox program. But if you need a sweetener and for some reason stevia or erythritol (aka Swerve) just won't cut it, raw local honey or manuka honey (which comes from bees that feed on the flowers of the manuka tree that's native to New Zealand and Australia) is your only good choice. The enzymes in honey do provide it some health benefit that no other natural sugar can match.

Inulin: Sold under the brand name Just Like Sugar, inulin is made from chicory root or agave (the plant used to make tequila, not the sweetener) and is useful in baking and in regular cooking as a replacement for sugar. It provides your gut buddies with a polysaccharide that they love but you can't digest. You can also find it at Whole Foods under the brand name Viv Agave Organic Blue Agave Inulin, or online.

Millet: You're probably familiar with millet as it is a popular component of birdseed. But it is not just for the birds! This hull-less (and thus, lectin-free) grain is a tasty addition to your diet.

Miracle Rice: If you're really missing your rice and eating a small amount of white basmati rice just isn't going to cut it—and you don't want to burn out on cauliflower rice—look for Miracle Rice in the refrigerated section, near the tofu. It's made from konjac root, which is lectin-free.

Mozzarella: True mozzarella—the kind that comes in ball-shapes of different sizes—is made from the milk of water buffalo, meaning it doesn't have casein A1. Read the label carefully; you want to buy "buffalo mozzarella." Chances are, if the mozzarella is shredded, it's made with cow's milk. You can also find goat's milk mozzarella, but you may have to go to Whole Foods or Amazon to find it.

Nori: If you're missing the convenience of tortillas for wraps, try this seaweed product that is often used in sushi rolls and is about the thickness of a sheet of paper. It's great for scrambled eggs, tuna or salmon salad, or other sandwich fixings. Look for organic nori.

Nutritional yeast: This is not the kind of yeast that causes bread to rise; it's a B-vitamin-rich powder that lends a savory, cheesy taste to whatever you sprinkle it on. It's available in natural food stores or online.

Olive oil: I prefer European olive oils, especially Italian olive oil, but a great American olive oil is called "O." California Olive Ranch makes a reliable and affordable oil as well. Make sure to buy extra-virgin—I get mine at Costco; it comes from Tuscany in Italy. If you can find (and afford) organic, that's your best choice. Good olive oil should be noticeably green, have a fresh, grassy smell, and come in an opaque glass bottle because it is photosensitive. By the way, if it makes you cough when you first try it, buy it! That means it has a lot of polyphenols.

Paprika: Another pepper-derived spice, like cayenne pepper, that doesn't include the skins and seeds and is therefore low-lectin. It imparts a rich flavor to a variety of dishes, particularly the smoked varieties.

Parmigiano-Reggiano: The real deal Parmesan cheese, made from the milk of Italian cows—which don't have casein A1 in their milk—harvested only during the spring and fall when grasses are abundant (meaning the cows are grass-fed). It can cost up to $20 per pound, but a little bit of this strong, salty cheese packs a big punch. Hold on to the rinds and add them to your broths, stocks, and soups for even more depth of flavor.

Pecorino-Romano: This Tuscan grating cheese is made from sheep's milk, making it a good fit for the Plant Paradox program.

Perilla oil: This oil, made from the seeds of the perilla plant, is low lectin and the most common cooking oil used in most Asian countries. It is a great source of the omega-3 fat alpha linolenic acid—containing more of it than any other oil, with the added benefit of having brain-boosting rosmarinic acid in it. Because perilla oil is a bit harder to find—look for it in Asian markets, natural food stores, and Whole Foods—I don't call for it in the recipes in this book, but it can be used interchangeably with olive oil or coconut oil.

Quorn products: This is a meat substitute derived from mushroom "roots," although it doesn't taste as "meaty" as your typical mushroom; it's more similar in taste and texture to chicken. Not all Quorn products are Plant Paradox–friendly—stick to the tenders, cutlets, and ground versions. It's important to note that these products aren't vegan—there's a little egg white protein in them. The products in the vegan line contain potato and gluten, so they aren't part of the Plant Paradox program. Stay away from any breaded version. You can find Quorn products in the vegetarian freezer section of most supermarkets.

Sea salt, iodized: Sea salt contains many more trace minerals than traditional table salt and is therefore much more healthful. However, be sure to look for versions of sea salt that contain added iodine. Iodine is essential to thyroid function, and the most typical way we get it is by eating iodized table salt. Once the foodie craze kicked in and so many people switched to sea salt, which typically *isn't* iodized, we started to see iodine deficiencies become more common. So give yourself the best of both worlds and buy iodized sea salt. It's pretty easy to find in most supermarkets, and even Morton's now has an iodized sea salt.

How to Reduce the Lectin Content of Your Favorite Foods

Once you're in Phase 3 of the Plant Paradox program, you can start eating some foods that contain lectins again—so long as you don't notice any adverse reactions, such as achiness, brain fog, or digestive issues. Knowing how to prepare your foods will help reduce the overall lectin content. To that end, here's a handy guide to how to do that.

FOOD	PREPARATION	COOKING
TOMATOES	Peel and seed—a serrated vegetable peeler makes this easy, or you can core them, cut a shallow X across the bottom and then pop them in boiling water for 30 seconds to loosen the skins.	Pressure-cooking your tomato soup or tomato sauce will reduce the lectin content even further.
PEPPERS	Removing the skins and seeds of your favorite peppers (whether big bell peppers or smaller chili peppers) removes most of their lectins. Again, a serrated peeler comes in handy here.	Roasting peppers—either on a grill, directly on a gas burner, or under a broiler in the oven—makes the skins easy to remove. Fermenting also reduces lectins, and most hot sauces are fermented.
ZUCCHINI AND EGGPLANTS	Technically fruits because they contain seeds, these foods have a lower lectin level when you eat the baby versions (which have fewer seeds). Peeling them will reduce lectins even further.	Pressure-cooking destroys the lectins present in these nightshades and renders the flesh of the plants tender and moist for use in pasta dishes.
BEANS	Soaking beans in plenty of water with multiple water changes over 24 to 48 hours before cooking reduces lectins.	Pressure-cooking destroys whatever lectins remain. If you don't have a pressure cooker, look for Eden Brand beans; they are pressure-cooked right in their cans.

FOOD	PREPARATION	COOKING
RICE	Because lectins are contained mostly in the brown hull that covers grains of rice, white rice has fewer lectins than brown rice. Rinsing the rice before you cook it also helps. Because Indian basmati rice has the highest resistant starch content of any rice, I recommend you stick to small amounts of that version if you choose to eat rice. To further increase the resistant starch of rice, refrigerate it after cooking, then reheat when ready to use.	Pressure-cooking rice reduces lectins further.
CUCUMBERS, SQUASHES, MELONS, PEACHES, AND OTHER FRUITS	Two words: Peel and seed.	
SOY	Fermenting removes most of the lectins from soybeans, which means that the fermented forms of soy, including miso, tempeh (the grain-free kind), and natto are preferable to tofu and edamame.	

Sorghum: Along with millet, sorghum is one of the very rare grains without a hull and thus is a lectin-free grain. It can be eaten as a breakfast cereal, served as a side dish, or even popped like popcorn. Bob's Red Mill carries it, or you can find a popped version of it, called Mini Pops, online.

Stevia: This natural sweetener contains no calories and won't cause a spike in blood sugar. Derived from the stevia plant, you can buy it in powdered form or in liquid drops. Because it is 300 times sweeter than sugar, a little goes quite a long way. I prefer the SweetLeaf brand because it doesn't have fillers such as maltodextrin like other brands often do, and the first ingredient is inulin, which your gut buddies love.

Tempeh: Tempeh is a form of fermented soy that's sold in the refrigerator case by the tofu. Look for organic, non-GMO versions, as most soy is GMO, made without grains (most tempeh sold in the U.S. is mixed with grains). Like tofu, tempeh doesn't have a great taste on its own, but picks up the flavors of other ingredients well, and is a good source of protein for vegans and vegetarians.

Vanilla extract: Be careful to buy only vanilla extract that says "pure" on the label—otherwise, what you're buying likely contains a slew of chemicals that mimic the taste of vanilla rather than the beans themselves. If you are missing sweetened, flavored yogurts, add a touch of pure vanilla extract and a few drops of stevia to your goat, sheep, hemp, or coconut yogurt—even kids love it.

VeganEgg: Made from algal flour, nutritional yeast, and other plant sources, this product provides much of the same taste and binding abilities of real eggs. It is gluten-free, lectin-free, dairy-free, and non-GMO. This is a relatively new product from the makers of Vegenaise, so it's not widely available in stores yet, although you can buy it online at Thrive Market or Amazon.

Yogurt: You want to avoid most commercial yogurts for two important reasons—most of the cow's milk used to make it contains casein A1, and any flavored yogurt is loaded with added sugars and often artificial stabilizers and flavorings. Instead, stick to yogurt made from goat, sheep, hemp, or coconut milk. They are available at Whole Foods, Trader Joe's, and natural food grocery stores.

Kitchen Tools

Really all you need to cook the Plant Paradox way are a couple of knives, a few pans, and an oven. But having a handful of other tools on hand will make the process more enjoyable and your results even more delicious, both of which mean you'll be more likely to stick with it. These are the ones I use most often and recommend you consider purchasing if you don't have them already:

Blender: I use a blender nearly every day. The high-speed blenders on the market, such as Blendtec, Vitamix, or Ninja, make quick work of smoothies, can blend and heat soups (so no need to dirty a pan), and do some of your prep work for you by chopping and combining ingredients. If you don't have a full-size blender and don't want to acquire one, the Magic Bullet or the larger NutriBullet are good, smaller options.

Food processor: A food processor is like having three extra sets of hands. It chops, mixes, and slices in just a few pulses. And you'll never again have to scrape down the sides of a blender when making pesto!

Knives: Having a good chef's knife and paring knife makes prep work a breeze. Keep them well-sharpened as you are more likely to injure yourself with a dull knife than a sharp one. Good knives are a cook's best friend.

Magic Bullet: This mini appliance is a blender/food processor hybrid. And because it's inexpensive, it's a great starter blender. The only drawback is that it is small. If you cook for a family or regularly entertain, you would probably be better served with a full-size high-speed blender.

Microwave: You probably already have one and if you don't, you certainly don't need to purchase one in order to be able to make these recipes. But if you do have one, you can get a few meals in this book on the table in minutes.

Mixing bowls: These are the type of kitchen tools where having the right ones makes a huge difference in your ease and enjoyment. Look for a set of mixing bowls (large, medium, and small) with high sides so the contents don't slosh over the edge and onto your counter or floor. You could use a stand mixer in lieu of mixing bowls—if you have a stand mixer, it may come in handy when making the recipes in this book—though I mixed every recipe myself by hand. (I didn't want to lug my stand mixer out from the bottom shelf, and I liked knowing that recipes could be done by hand if you don't happen to have a stand mixer.)

Pressure cooker: If you want to enjoy eating beans or tomato sauce, a pressure cooker is invaluable. I love the Instant Pot, which is an electric pressure cooker that regulates the pressure for you, so you don't have to worry about potential explosions—a hazard of old-fashioned pressure cookers that you may recall from your grandmother's pressure-cooking days. You can also use an Instant Pot as a slow cooker, or as a sauté pan (it has a high-heat setting so you can brown meat or onions right in it without starting on the stove). I find them to be more than worth the expense—they cost about $100—but they also go on sale every Black Friday, and frequently you'll find them at Costco or Target for as little as $69. Just be sure never to overfill any type of pressure cooker, digital or not. That "do not fill above this line" line is not a suggestion, it's for your safety.

Salad spinner: I know what you might be thinking—*not another gadget!* But greens are such an important part of any healthy diet, and if they are dried properly they will last longer in the fridge and dressings will cling perfectly to them. I could not believe the difference this gadget made in my and my wife Penny's lives when we bought one! It makes buying organic greens and lettuces whole a snap to prepare: chop, throw in the spinner basket, rinse, then spin away the water! No more plastic bags that use questionable chemicals to keep that pre-chopped lettuce "fresh" for a week.

Skillets: Having a good pan makes food taste better and cleanup easier. Please resist the temptation to buy or use a skillet with a nonstick coating, as these are made out endocrine-disrupting chemicals that get released into your food. Instead, look for a skillet with a ceramic coating or high-quality stainless steel. And please, throw that cast iron skillet without a ceramic coating in the trash. I can't tell you the number of patients I see who use a cast iron skillet about once a week and have dangerously high iron levels.

Spiralizer: This handy tool makes noodles out of all kinds of vegetables, such as jicama, sweet potatoes, and daikon radish, so you can have a pasta-like dish that doesn't disrupt your gut. You don't need a fancy, electronic one. The hand-held version works just great and only costs about $15.

Vegetable peelers: Remember, lectins are found in the peels and seeds of plants, so having a peeler helps you lighten your lectin load. I recommend having two kinds: one with straight-edge blades and one with serrated-edge blades. The serrated edge lets you peel delicate things, like tomatoes, saving you the step of blanching them.

I'm not suggesting you need to invest in new kitchen gear, but even if you decide to buy one or two things, keep this in mind: The vast majority of my patients tell me that they save money on the Plant Paradox program. No more takeout or expensive prepared foods—just simple, whole foods. Not to mention the money they save when they throw out their prescriptions (with a doctor's supervision, of course).

And with that, let's get cooking!

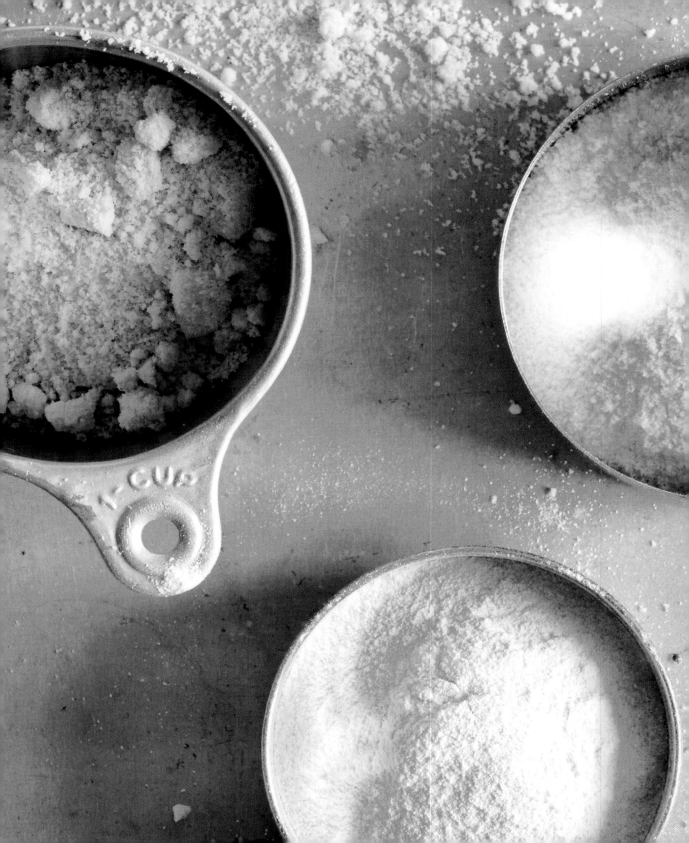

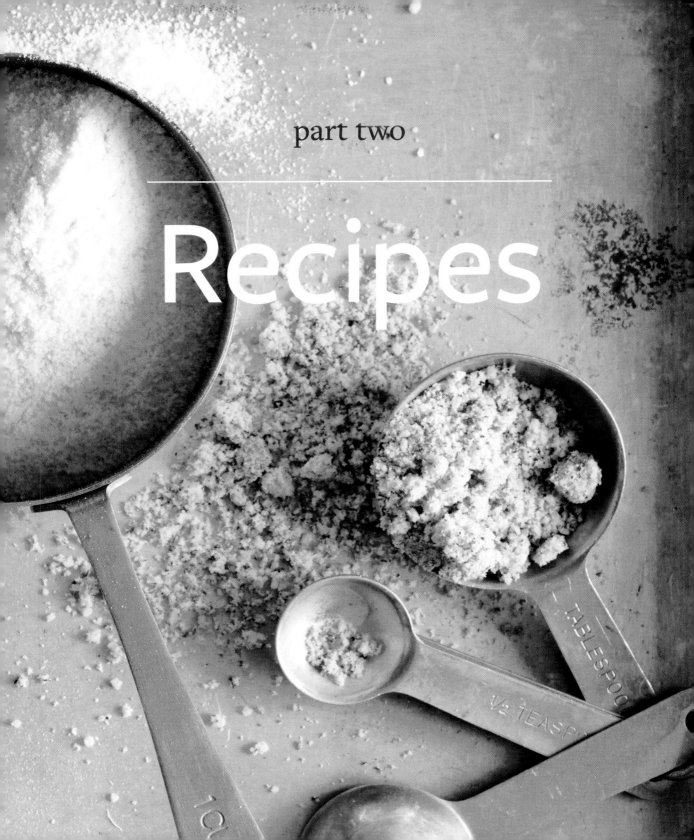

part two

Recipes

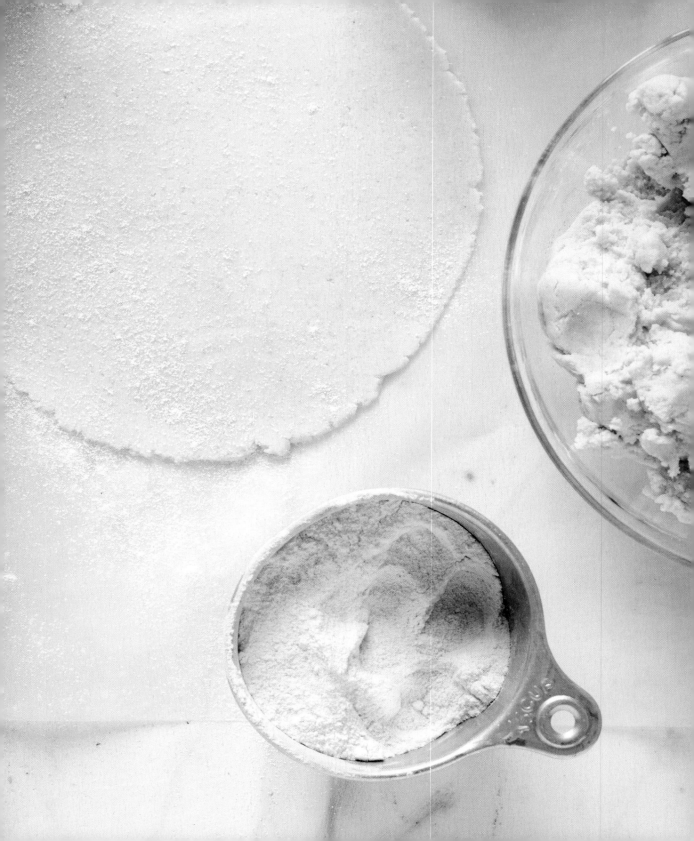

Appetizers and Snacks

Brazilian Cheesy Bread

There's a tiny neighborhood pizza place in Los Angeles that serves the most addictive Pão de Queijo—a super-flavorful Brazilian cheesy bread that fits the Plant Paradox program perfectly. If you've ever made cream puffs, this twice-cooked dough technique may be already familiar to you. It takes a little bit of extra time, but the results are worth it!

MAKES 24 2-INCH ROLLS

1 cup goat's milk, casein A2 milk, or unsweetened coconut milk

½ cup avocado oil

1 teaspoon iodized sea salt

10 ounces (about 2 cups) cassava flour

2 large omega-3 or pastured eggs or VeganEggs

1 to 1½ cups grated Parmigiano-Reggiano cheese, or 1 cup nutritional yeast

1. Arrange two racks in your oven so they're evenly spaced, and preheat the oven to 450°F.

2. Line two baking sheets with parchment paper or silicone baking mats.

3. Place the milk, oil, and salt in a medium saucepan. Bring to a simmer over medium heat, stirring occasionally. Remove from heat when big bubbles start to form.

4. Add the cassava flour to the saucepan and stir with a wooden spoon until mixture is well combined. A gelatinous dough will begin to form.

5. Transfer the dough into the bowl of a stand mixer fitted with the paddle attachment. Beat the dough for a few minutes at medium speed until it appears smooth, and is cool enough that you can touch it comfortably.*

6. Keeping the mixer on medium speed, beat the eggs into the cooled mixture one at a time. Wait until the first egg is fully incorporated before adding the second. Scrape down sides of the bowl regularly to ensure consistent mixing.

7. If using cheese, beat it in on medium speed. You'll end up with a stretchy, sticky dough that's softer than a cookie dough, but stiffer than a cake batter.

8. Scoop the dough with a small ice cream scoop and place on the baking sheets, spacing them evenly (you should

* If you don't have a stand mixer like a KitchenAid, that's okay. You can beat this dough by hand, but be prepared for a workout—10 to 15 minutes of vigorous beating, at least.

have about 12 per sheet). Dip scoop in a bowl of water between scoops to keep dough from sticking.

9. Place the baking sheets in the oven and reduce heat to 350°F. Bake for 15 minutes, then rotate the baking sheets.

10. Bake for an additional 10 to 15 minutes, until bread is golden. Remove from oven and cool for a few minutes before serving.

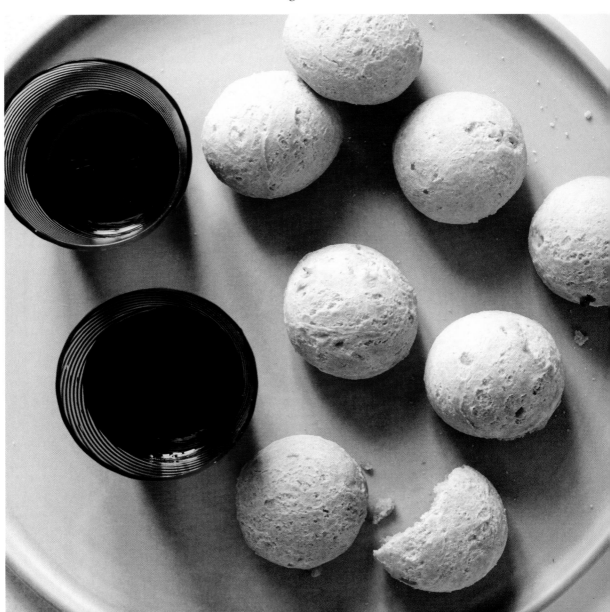

Avocado Deviled Eggs

Deviled eggs are a dinner party classic that make for a quick, easy appetizer, a really good snack, or even an on-the-go breakfast. These eggs taste just like the version you grew up with—except they're green! That's because I've swapped out the mayo and replaced it with creamy avocado. Packed with protein and good-for-you fats, this healthy, simple snack comes together in minutes.

MAKES 12

6 omega-3 or pastured eggs, hard-boiled and peeled

1 ripe avocado, skin and seed removed

1 tablespoon Dijon mustard

1 teaspoon grated horseradish

1 teaspoon iodized sea salt

Juice of 1 lemon

Paprika, to garnish

1. Cut the eggs in half lengthwise and remove the yolks, placing them in the work bowl of a food processor.

2. Add avocado, mustard, horseradish, sea salt, and lemon juice to the food processor bowl.* Blend until smooth.

3. Spoon the yolk mixture back into the egg whites, and garnish with a sprinkle of paprika.

If you don't have a food processor, place ingredients in a mixing bowl and mash with a fork or a potato masher until smooth.

Dr. Gundry's Nut Mix 2.0

When *The Plant Paradox* came out, people went crazy for the nut mix. So I thought, why not take it to the next level, and really give them something to talk about? By adding some of the healthiest ingredients on earth—like olive oil, garlic, and plenty of rosemary—we've taken this simple snack to new heights.

SERVES 12 TO 15

1 cup raw walnuts

1 cup raw pistachios

½ cup raw pecans

½ cup raw macadamia nuts

2 tablespoons extra-virgin olive oil

2 cloves garlic, minced

2 tablespoons fresh rosemary, minced

1 teaspoon paprika

1 teaspoon iodized sea salt

1. Combine nuts in a large bowl and set aside.

2. Heat olive oil in a small sauté pan over medium heat. Add garlic and rosemary, and cook until very fragrant, 2 to 3 minutes.

3. Remove from heat and pour oil mixture over nut mix immediately, then add paprika and sea salt.

4. Toss to combine and serve.

Cauliflower Fritters

These tasty fritters were inspired by a recipe from Sylvie Shirazi on her food blog Gourmande in the Kitchen. Where Sylvie uses broccoli, I use cauliflower. This is an exciting introduction to cauliflower for people who think they hate it, or another tasty way for cauliflower addicts to get their fix.

SERVES 4

FOR THE FRITTERS

7 ounces (approximately 2 cups) cauliflower florets, steamed until tender

2 large omega-3 or pastured eggs or VeganEggs

2 tablespoons coconut yogurt

2 green onions, finely chopped

1 tablespoon chopped parsley

1 tablespoon chopped mint

1 garlic clove, finely grated

2 tablespoons grated Parmesan cheese or nutritional yeast

5 to 6 tablespoons cassava flour

2 tablespoons coconut flour

¼ teaspoon baking soda

1 teaspoon iodized sea salt

⅛ teaspoon ground black pepper

3 to 4 tablespoons coconut oil, for frying

FOR THE YOGURT SAUCE

6 ounces coconut yogurt

2 tablespoons extra-virgin olive oil

1 tablespoon tahini

Juice of ½ lemon

1 teaspoon paprika

Pinch of iodized sea salt

1. In the work bowl of a food processor fitted with an S-blade, pulse the cauliflower, eggs, yogurt, green onion, parsley, mint, and garlic until finely crumbled and well combined.

2. Transfer to a mixing bowl, then add the cheese or yeast and 2 tablespoons of cassava flour, coconut flour, baking soda, salt, and pepper, and mix again. The mixture should form a cohesive dough. If it's too runny, add more cassava flour, one teaspoon at a time.

3. Let the mixture rest for 5 minutes—the perfect opportunity to make the yogurt sauce.

4. Whisk together the yogurt, olive oil, tahini, lemon juice, paprika, and sea salt. Set aside until ready to serve.

5. Heat the coconut oil in a medium skillet over medium heat.

6. Spoon a tablespoon of batter in the pan. Flatten with the back of a spoon or spatula until approximately fritter-shaped. Cook for 2 minutes per side, flipping carefully. Do no more than three or four fritters at a time to prevent the pan from crowding.

7. Cook in batches until all the batter is used. Serve the fritters fresh out of the skillet with the yogurt sauce on the side.

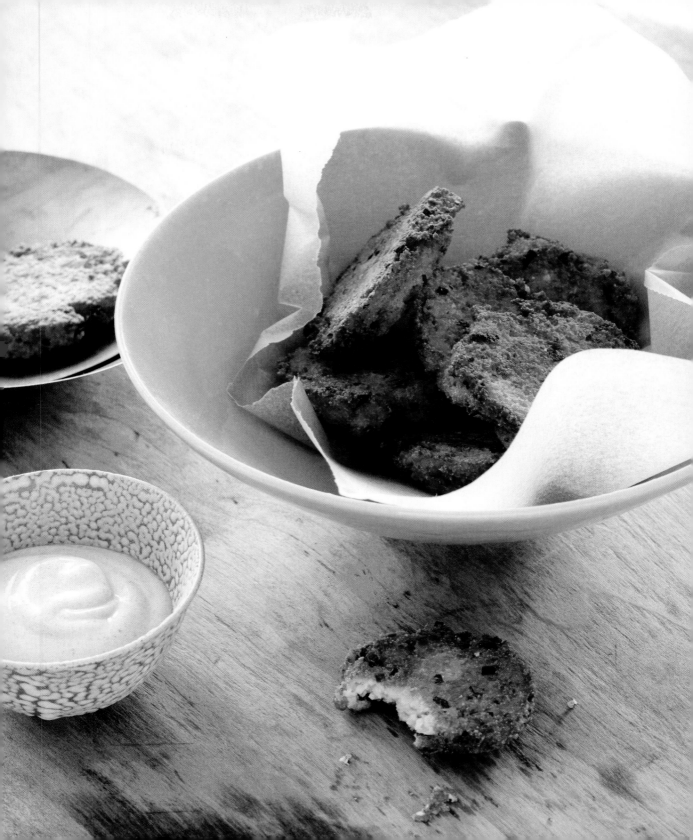

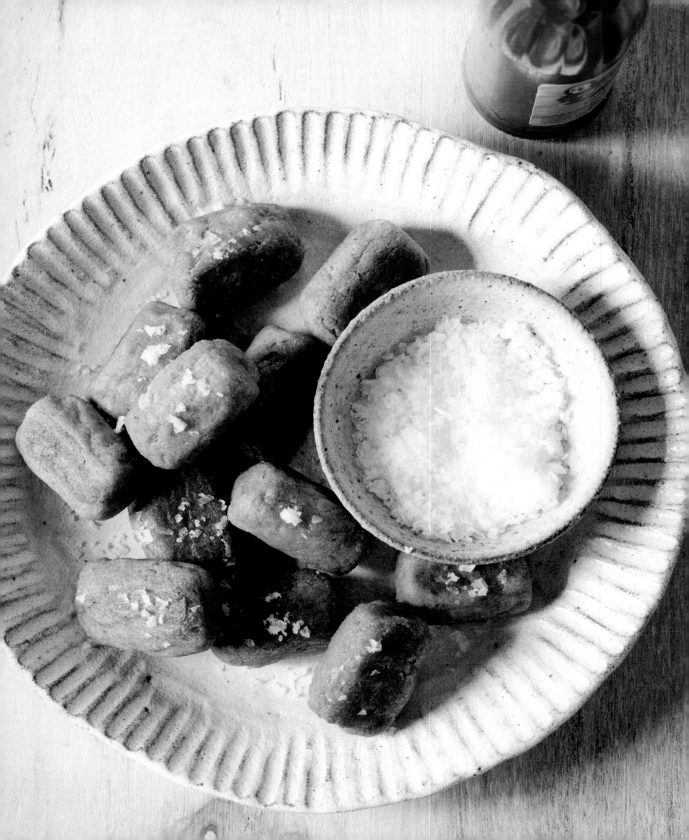

Broccoli Puffs

If you're hooked on tater tots, or just love finger food, these broccoli puffs are an easy twist on the classic. As a bonus, they're a great way to use up any leftover steamed broccoli you may have in your fridge. Try them dipped in hot sauce or guacamole, or serve them as "croutons" on your favorite soup.

MAKES ABOUT 20

2 cups broccoli florets, steamed until tender

1 egg or VeganEgg

½ yellow onion, minced

1 clove garlic, minced

½ cup cassava flour

¼ cup blanched almond meal

½ teaspoon black pepper

½ teaspoon yacón syrup or local honey

1 teaspoon iodized sea salt

1 tablespoon minced parsley

¼ cup grated Parmigiano-Reggiano cheese or nutritional yeast

Hot sauce or Plant Paradox Guacamole (page 259), for dipping (optional)

1. Preheat the oven to 400°F. Grease a baking sheet with a thin layer of oil and set aside.

2. In the work bowl of a food processor fitted with an S-blade,* pulse the broccoli, egg, onion, garlic, cassava flour, almond meal, pepper, syrup or honey, salt, parsley, and cheese or yeast.

3. Scoop about one and a half tablespoons of mix and gently press between your hands to form a tater-tot shape. Wash your hands between every few tots to prevent sticking. Place the tots on the baking sheet, evenly spaced.

4. Bake for about 18 to 20 minutes, or until golden brown. Serve with hot sauce or guacamole if desired.

It's fine to use a high-speed blender, like a VitaMix, too. Just work in batches, taking care not to overfill, because the mixture can get stuck in the bottom and get over-blended and turn mushy.

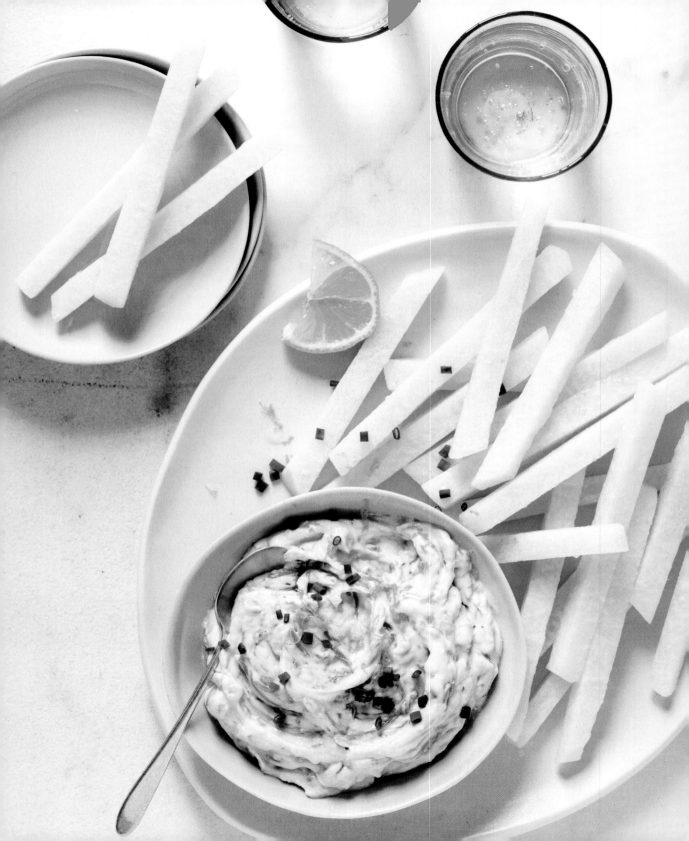

Caramelized Onion Dip

A healthy take on the comfort-food classic, this dip has all the addictive sweet and savory flavors of traditional onion dip—but it's actually *good* for you. You can pair this dip with any of the chips in this chapter, but my favorite way to serve it is with fresh, crispy jicama sticks.

SERVES 6 TO 8

2 tablespoons extra-virgin olive oil

2 large yellow onions, thinly sliced

1 clove garlic, minced

1 tablespoon fresh thyme leaves

1 teaspoon fresh rosemary, minced

1 teaspoon iodized sea salt

1 teaspoon ground black pepper

Zest of 1 lemon

Juice of 1 lemon

2 cups plain coconut yogurt

Minced chives, to garnish

1 jicama, peeled and cut into sticks.

1. Heat the olive oil in a large pan over medium-low heat. Add the onions and cook, stirring regularly, until onions are tender and translucent, about 8 minutes.

2. Add garlic, thyme, rosemary, sea salt, pepper, and lemon zest, and continue to cook, stirring regularly until onions are evenly browned, about 10 to 15 minutes. (If garlic starts to brown, reduce heat to low.)

3. Stir in the lemon juice, then remove the pan from heat and let cool to room temperature.

4. Place the coconut yogurt in a bowl and stir in the cooled onion mixture until combined. Transfer dip to serving dish and garnish with chives. Serve with jicama sticks, other fresh veggies, chips, or crackers.

Cassava Tortillas (and Chips)

No one wants to give up chips and guacamole . . . and on the Plant Paradox plan, you don't have to. These tortillas work better as a flatbread or for tacos than as wraps, but they really shine when baked into chips—the perfect accompaniment to guacamole.

MAKES 10 LARGE OR 18 SMALL TORTILLAS

2 cups cassava flour

1 cup unsweetened coconut milk or goat's milk

½ cup avocado oil

½ cup water

2 teaspoons iodized sea salt

Olive oil, ghee, or avocado oil, for cooking

TO MAKE TORTILLAS

1. In a medium bowl, combine the cassava flour, milk, avocado oil, salt, and water. Mix together with a wooden spoon until well combined. The dough should have a smooth, cohesive consistency.

2. Divide the dough into 10 larger or 18 smaller equal parts and shape into balls. On a piece of parchment paper, use a rolling pin to roll each section into a slightly thicker than average tortilla. (If you have a tortilla press, feel free to use it instead.) If dough sticks to the rolling pin, sprinkle it with a light dusting of cassava flour.

3. Heat a frying pan on the stove over medium-low heat. Brush pan with oil or ghee, then cook the tortillas for 3 to 4 minutes each side (depending on how crisp or soft you like them).

4. Serve immediately unless making into chips.

TO MAKE CHIPS

1. Preheat the oven to 425°F. Brush a sheet tray with oil and set aside.

2. Brush both sides of tortillas with avocado oil, and cut into chip-size wedges.

3. Arrange in a single layer on the baking sheet and bake for 10 to 15 minutes, until crispy.

4. Serve with Plant Paradox Guacamole (page 259).

NOTE: *These are not as easy to handle as flour tortillas—they're rather delicate. So take care in transferring them to the pan and flipping them, as they tend to crack. I find it's easier to make small tortillas until you get used to handling this delicate dough.*

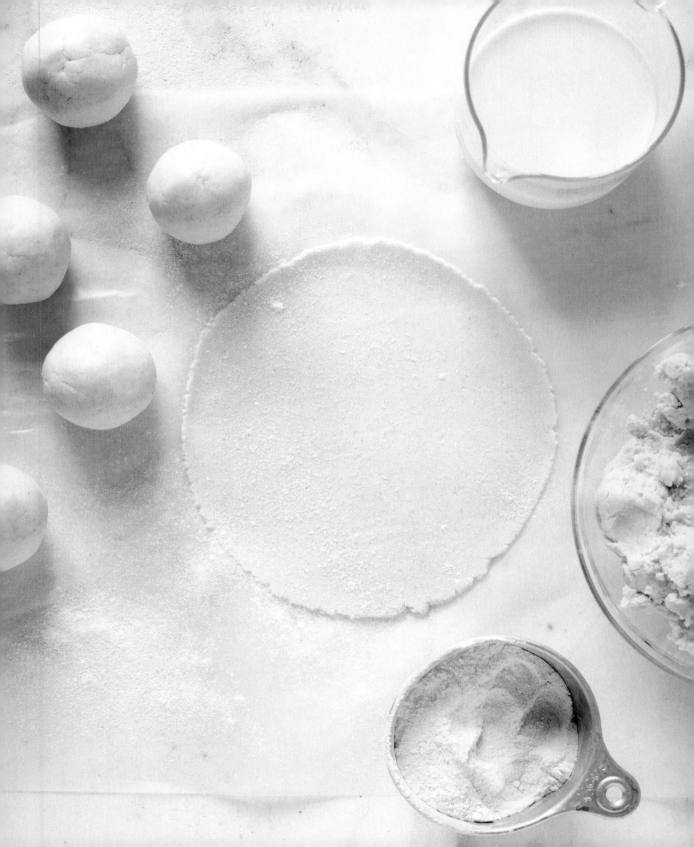

Chips Three Ways

When people start on the Plant Paradox plan, they often complain about missing snack foods like chips. But I want people to feel empowered, not deprived. So I worked with my friend Irina Skoeries, the founder of Catalyst Cuisine, to develop not one, but three different chip recipes to scratch that junk food itch in a healthy way!

Sweet Potato Chips

1 Japanese sweet potato, peeled

2 to 3 cups avocado oil or extra-virgin olive oil

2 tablespoons iodized sea salt

1. Using a vegetable peeler, slice the sweet potato into thin slices.

2. Coat the bottom of a large skillet with 1 to 2 inches of oil.

3. Heat oil on medium until "shimmering."

4. Sear the sweet potato slices until golden brown on one side. Flip and repeat.

5. Place the golden chips on a paper towel and sprinkle with salt.

6. Repeat the process until all slices are golden brown.

Plantain Chips

2 green plantains, peeled and thinly sliced

1½ tablespoons olive oil

¾ teaspoon salt

Freshly ground pepper to taste

1. Preheat the oven to 400°F. Place parchment paper on a cookie sheet and set aside.

2. In a bowl, combine plantain slices, olive oil, and seasonings by gently tossing with your hands.

3. Spread plantains on prepared cookie sheet in a single layer.

4. Bake for 15 to 20 minutes, turning plantains halfway through (after about 8 minutes).

5. Remove from the oven when plantain chips start to brown around the edges.

Prosciutto Chips

10 thin slices pasture-raised prosciutto

1. Preheat the oven to 350°F. Place parchment paper on a cookie sheet.

2. Lay the slices of prosciutto on the parchment-lined cookie sheet in a single layer.

3. Bake until crispy, about 5 to 7 minutes. Leave them to cool (they get crispier when chilled).

4. Break into smaller pieces, and add them to any entrée as a topping, on top of salads, or just eat them by themselves. Watch out—they are very addictive!

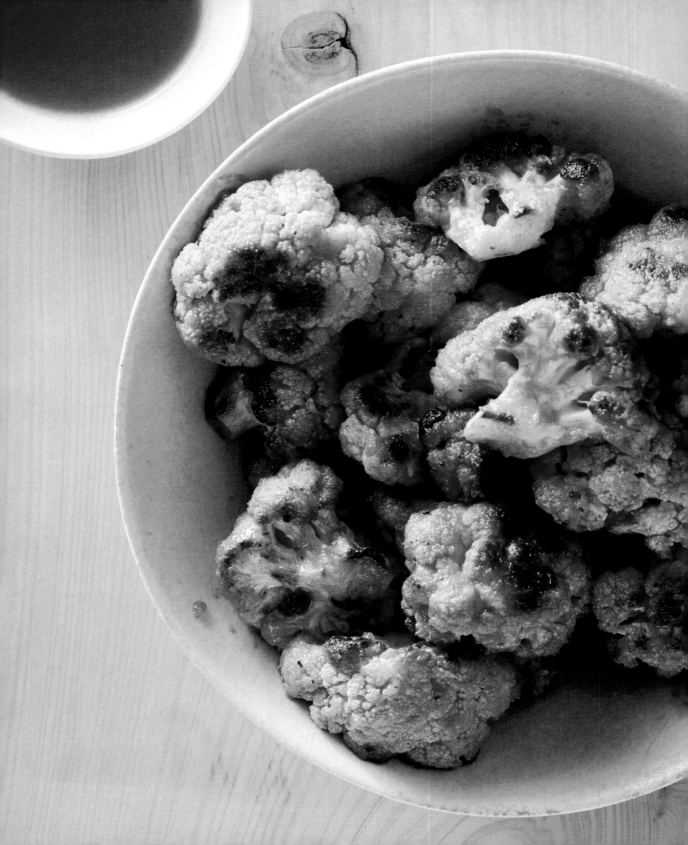

Buffalo Cauliflower Bites

There's nothing like settling into a plate of spicy, tangy wings while watching a game. But let's be honest—the sauce is usually better than the chicken! In my Plant Paradox–approved version, you can still enjoy the addictive flavor and crunch of your favorite game day treat—without the halftime stomachache!

SERVES 4 TO 6

FOR THE BUFFALO SAUCE

½ cup Frank's Red Hot Sauce

2½ teaspoons avocado oil or ghee

1 tablespoon coconut aminos

1 teaspoon apple cider vinegar

1 medium head of cauliflower, chopped

2 tablespoons extra-virgin olive oil, plus more for baking sheet

2 tablespoons cassava flour

1 teaspoon iodized sea salt

1 teaspoon ground black pepper

2 teaspoons garlic powder

½ cup buffalo sauce (recipe above)

Plain coconut yogurt, for dipping

1. Preheat the oven to 450°F.

2. First, make the buffalo sauce: combine the hot sauce, avocado oil or ghee, coconut aminos, and apple cider vinegar in a glass jar with a lid and shake well. Refrigerate until needed.

3. Drizzle a baking sheet liberally with olive oil, or line with parchment. Set aside.

4. Toss the cauliflower, olive oil, cassava flour, and spices together in a large bowl until cauliflower is evenly coated.

5. Transfer to a baking sheet and bake for 30 minutes, turning every 10 minutes so the cauliflower crisps on all sides.

6. Brush with the buffalo sauce, then bake an additional 10 minutes.

7. Serve with yogurt and any extra buffalo sauce for dipping.

Garlic-and-Walnut-Stuffed Mushrooms

Stuffed mushrooms were always a dinner party favorite at my house, but a stuffing made of sausage and rice just doesn't cut it on the Plant Paradox plan. These days I make my stuffed mushrooms with walnuts, plenty of garlic, and onions—and I like them even better! If you enjoy a little bit of heat, add a dash of hot sauce when you stir in the coconut cream.

SERVES 12

12 bite-size brown mushrooms, such as cremini, wiped with a damp towel

¼ cup plus 2 tablespoons extra-virgin olive oil

½ brown onion, minced

4 cloves garlic

1 teaspoon fresh thyme

1 cup diced walnuts

½ teaspoon salt

½ teaspoon poultry seasoning

½ teaspoon paprika

¼ cup coconut cream

¼ cup minced parsley, to garnish (optional)

1. Prepare the mushrooms by removing the stems. Crumble stems and set aside.

2. Heat 2 tablespoons of olive oil in a large skillet with a lid. When oil is shimmering, cook onions, garlic, thyme, and reserved mushroom stems over medium-high heat until tender.

3. Add the walnuts, salt, poultry seasoning, and paprika, and sauté until fragrant.

4. Remove from heat and whisk in coconut cream.

5. Spoon the mixture into the mushrooms, packing them tightly.

6. Heat the remaining olive oil in a skillet with a cover over medium heat.

7. Cook stuffed mushrooms, stuffed side up, over medium heat for 2 to 3 minutes.

8. Reduce heat to low, cover, and cook an additional 10 to 15 minutes until tender. Serve garnished with parsley, if desired.

Grain-Free Crackers*

These delicious (and really versatile) crackers will soon become a staple in your pantry. This technique might feel a little tricky at first, but with practice you'll be a pro in no time. I like to pair these with my Addictive Caramelized Onion Bourbon Jam (page 254) for a simple and elegant appetizer.

MAKES ABOUT 16 CRACKERS

1 cup blanched almond flour

¾ cups plus 1 tablespoon tapioca starch

2½ tablespoon arrowroot powder

1 teaspoon onion powder

1 teaspoon iodized sea salt

½ teaspoon white pepper

⅛ teaspoon xanthan gum

1 cup water (approximately)

¼ cup toppings of your choice

TOPPING IDEAS:

Everything: salt, poppy seeds, toasted onion flakes, and black toasted sesame seeds, or Trader Joe's "Everything But the Bagel" seasoning

Caraway seeds and salt

Fennel seeds and salt

Rosemary and salt

Parmigiano-Reggiano cheese

See page 255 for a photo of the finished product!

1. Preheat the oven to 350°F. Line baking sheet with silicone nonstick baking sheets (Silpats).

2. First, make the crackers: In a medium mixing bowl, combine the almond flour, tapioca starch, arrowroot, onion powder, salt, white pepper, and xanthan gum. Mix well with a whisk.

3. Slowly add the water to the mixture. You want the batter to resemble a thin pancake batter. If more water is needed, add and mix at this time.

4. Using a ¼-cup measuring cup or another utensil, carefully pour 3 rows of 4 circles of batter on the baking sheet. The circles should be approximately 2¾ inches to 3 inches across. (They will continue to spread a little after pouring.)

5. Sprinkle each cracker with desired topping.

6. Bake for 10 minutes at 350°F, then increase heat to 400°F. (Starting with the lower temperature helps prevent crackers from bubbling up in the center so they stay flat.)

7. Bake for another 20 minutes, or until crackers are golden. Transfer them to a cooling rack and, once cooled completely, store in an airtight container for up to 5 days. (Although they will lose their crispiness after day 2, they remain tasty.)

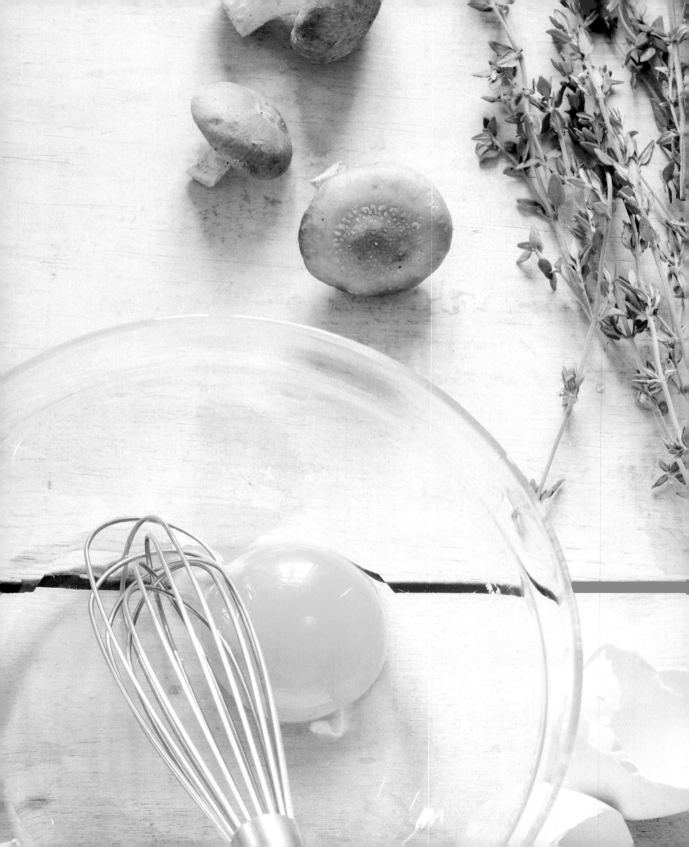

Morning Meals

Carrot Cake Muffins

Is there anything more tantalizing than the sweetly spiced flavor of carrot cake? Most versions are full of sugar and butter or canola oil, but this Plant Paradox–friendly recipe is sugar-free and packed with healthy fats. I like to make a big batch of these muffins and freeze half of them—that way, I've got a perfect breakfast or snack on hand anytime. Just defrost in the microwave for 30 seconds and enjoy!

MAKES 12 MUFFINS

1¼ cups blanched almond flour

2 tablespoons coconut flour

½ teaspoon baking soda

⅛ teaspoon salt

1½ teaspoons ground cinnamon

½ teaspoon ground ginger

¼ teaspoon ground nutmeg

2 omega-3 or pastured eggs or VeganEggs

⅓ cup MCT oil or avocado oil

⅔ cup unsweetened coconut milk

⅓ cup Swerve (erythritol)

2 teaspoons vanilla

2 large carrots, grated

¼ cup chopped walnuts

1. Preheat the oven to 350°F. Prepare a muffin tin with cupcake liners and set aside.

2. In a large bowl, whisk together the almond flour, coconut flour, baking soda, salt, cinnamon, ginger, and nutmeg.

3. In a small bowl, combine the eggs, oil, coconut milk, Swerve, and vanilla.

4. Whisk wet ingredients into dry, then add the grated carrots and walnuts.

5. Fold to combine.

6. Portion into the muffin tin, dividing mixture evenly among 12 cups.

7. Bake for 12 to 18 minutes, or until a toothpick inserted into the center of the muffins comes out clean. Allow muffins to cool slightly before serving. When stored in an airtight container, muffins will stay fresh 5 days in the refrigerator or 3 months in the freezer.

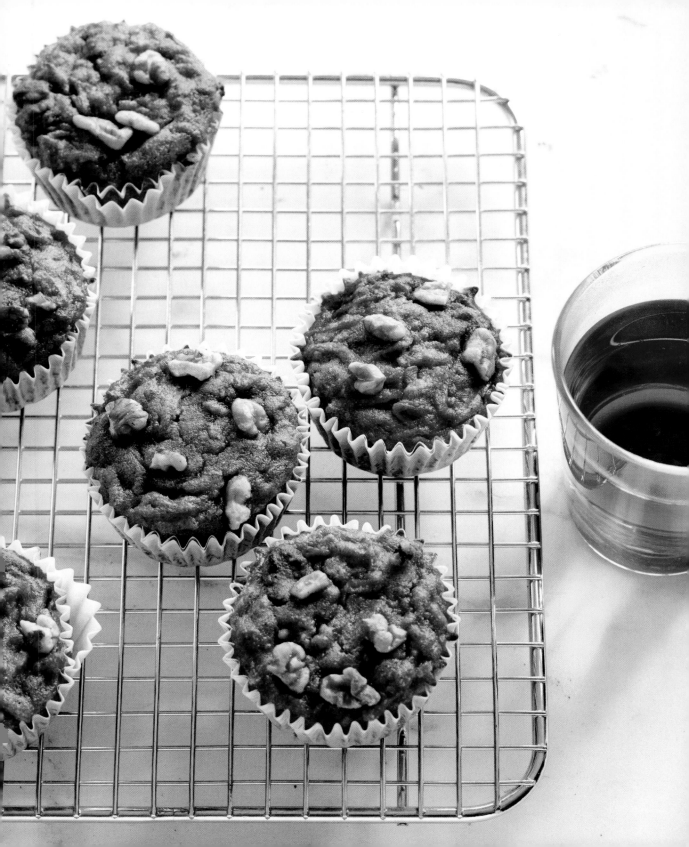

Caramelized Onion and Gruyère Quiche

Gruyère is famous for its delectable texture when melted, and is a key ingredient in cheese fondue. Best of all, because it is made from the milk of Southern European cows, it doesn't contain the lectin-like protein casein A1. In this recipe, the Gruyère melds perfectly with the eggs, mushrooms, and caramelized onions and elevates this dish to a supremely comforting, yet still healthy breakfast.

SERVES 6

1 Plant Paradox Piecrust (page 238)

2 tablespoons extra-virgin olive oil

1 medium yellow onion, thinly sliced

8 ounces sliced mixed mushrooms, like cremini, oyster, or shiitake

2 large pastured or omega-3 eggs or VeganEggs

2 large egg yolks, or 2 more Vegan Eggs

⅔ cup grated Gruyère cheese

1¼ cups goat's milk or coconut milk

¼ teaspoon iodized sea salt

¼ teaspoon white pepper

Pinch of fresh grated nutmeg (optional)

1. Preheat the oven to 375°F.

2. In a medium skillet, heat the oil and caramelize the onions by cooking low and slow, stirring frequently, until well browned. Add the sliced mushrooms toward the middle of cooking.

3. In a large mixing bowl, whisk the eggs and egg yolks together. Mix in the cheese, goat's or coconut milk, salt, white pepper, and nutmeg.

4. In pre-baked piecrust, pour in the mushrooms, onions and cheese. Distribute evenly, then pour the egg mixture on top. Sprinkle with nutmeg, if using.

5. Bake for approximately 30 to 35 minutes, until slightly toasted on top.

Ralph's Breakfast Scramble

Ralph first came to my office with his husband, Steve, who was experiencing a range of health issues that cleared up once he started following the Plant Paradox program. Both Ralph and Steve are excellent cooks and have supplied me with a steady stream of new recipes that are Plant Paradox–friendly, and now I'm excited to share some of them with you. Ralph created this recipe because he and Steve don't like starting the day with a sweet dish—it's a great, savory way to break your nightly fast.

SERVES 1 TO 2

1 tablespoon extra-virgin olive oil

½ medium onion, diced

½ teaspoon iodized sea salt

½ teaspoon paprika

3 omega-3 or pastured eggs or VeganEggs

¼ teaspoon pepper

½ teaspoon dried basil

½ teaspoon Mt. Hood Toasted Onion All Purpose Rub, or ½ teaspoon powdered onion

¼ teaspoon cayenne

½ ripe avocado, diced

1. Heat the olive oil in a medium or large skillet over low heat.

2. Add the onions, salt, and paprika into skillet and sauté for about 20 minutes, or until lightly caramelized.

3. As onions are caramelizing, in a medium bowl, add the eggs, a dash of salt, pepper, basil, Mt. Hood Toasted Onion Rub or onion powder, and cayenne. Mix well.

4. Cut the avocado into small squares, then add it to the egg mixture, stirring in lightly.

5. Pour the egg mixture into the same skillet you used for the onions and cook over medium heat. Scramble the eggs and remove from heat when they reach your desired taste and texture.

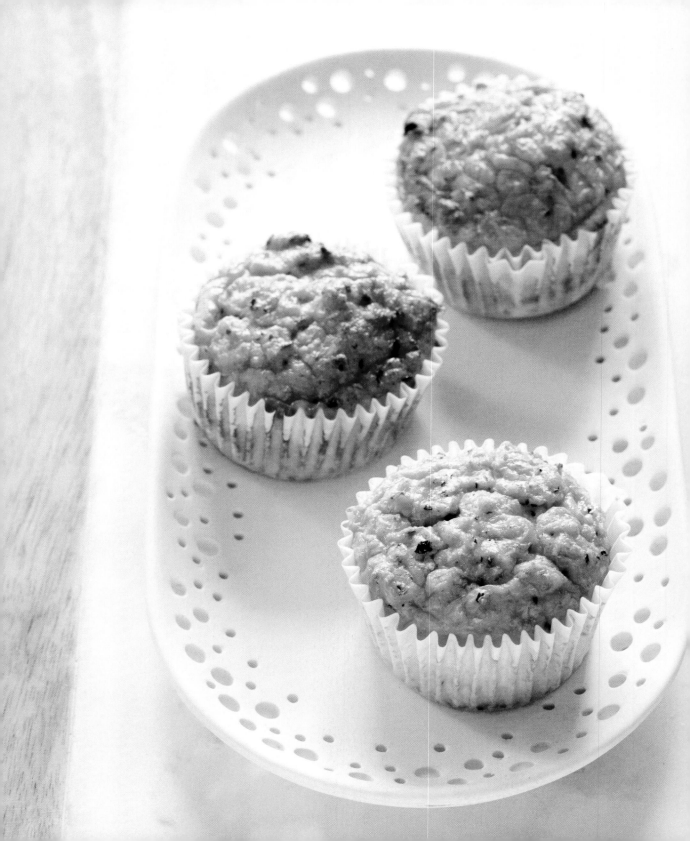

Cheesy Cauliflower Muffins

These muffins are a great grab-and-go option for busy mornings. They're savory, cheesy, eggy—all of the things that you crave in a quick breakfast bite. Top them with a little hot sauce for some extra kick!

MAKES 12 MUFFINS

1 tablespoon extra-virgin olive oil

3 cups cauliflower rice

½ teaspoon iodized sea salt

¼ teaspoon garlic powder

¼ teaspoon paprika

½ teaspoon dried basil

3 omega-3 or pastured eggs or VeganEggs

½ cup grated Parmigiano-Reggiano cheese or nutritional yeast

¼ cup cassava flour

½ teaspoon aluminum-free baking powder

Dash of hot sauce (optional)

1. Preheat the oven to 375°F. Prepare a muffin tin with cupcake liners and set aside.

2. Heat the olive oil in a sauté pan over medium-high heat. Add the cauliflower rice and sea salt and cook, stirring frequently, until cauliflower is tender, about 3 to 5 minutes.

3. Add garlic powder, paprika, and basil, and cook for an additional 2 minutes. Let cool to room temperature.

4. In a large bowl, combine the cauliflower mixture, eggs, and cheese or nutrional yeast.

5. In a small bowl, whisk together the cassava flour and baking powder.

6. Fold the dry ingredients into the cauliflower mix along with the hot sauce, then portion into muffin tins.

7. Bake for 20 to 25 minutes until no longer wet to the touch. Let cool at least 5 minutes before serving.

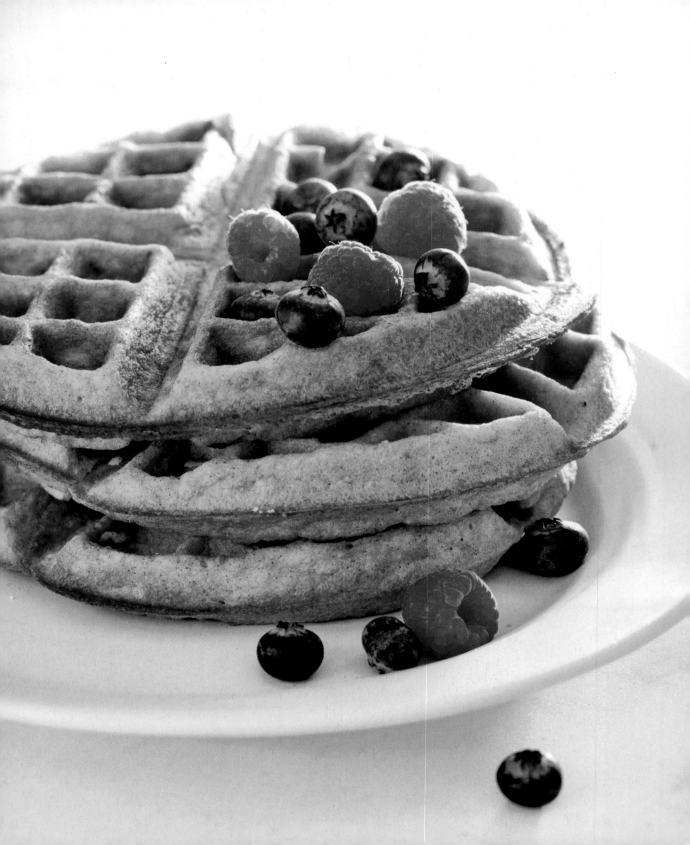

Coconut Macadamia Waffles

These waffles are an extra-special breakfast that folks of all ages love. They're sweet enough to eat on their own, but if you want an extra-decadent breakfast, top them with a little coconut cream. If you don't have a waffle iron, this recipe also works well as pancake batter.

SERVES 3 TO 4

4 tablespoons MCT oil or melted coconut oil, plus extra for waffle iron

4 omega-3 or pastured eggs or VeganEggs

⅔ cup unsweetened coconut milk

5 or 6 drops stevia

½ teaspoon vanilla extract

½ teaspoon iodized sea salt

½ teaspoon aluminum-free baking powder

¼ cup coconut flour

½ teaspoon cinnamon

¼ cup macadamia nuts, finely chopped

½ cup coconut cream, to serve

1. Preheat your waffle iron per manufacturer's instructions.

2. In a large bowl, whisk together the oil, eggs, coconut milk, stevia, and vanilla extract.

3. Add the dry ingredients to wet and whisk until thoroughly combined.

4. Fold in the macadamia nuts.

5. Use MCT or coconut oil to coat the waffle iron, then cook according to your model's instructions, approximately one-third of a cup batter per 4-inch square waffle.

6. Serve topped with coconut cream.

Chocolate Chip Mini-Pancakes

When you think about what constitutes a healthy breakfast, "chocolate" and "pancakes" are probably two of the last words that come to mind. But these gluten-free pancakes are low in sugar and packed with protein. The addition of high-cacao chocolate not only gives these pancakes a boost of antioxidants, magnesium, and iron . . . it also makes them taste a lot like dessert!

SERVES 3 TO 4 (MAKES 12 TO 14 MINI-PANCAKES)

6 omega-3 or pastured eggs or VeganEggs

1½ cups water

2 teaspoons almond extract

1 cup coconut flour

½ cup tapioca starch

½ cup arrowroot starch

2 tablespoons monk-fruit sweetener or 1 packet stevia

1 teaspoon baking powder

1 teaspoon baking soda

¼ teaspoon iodized sea salt

1 cup 85 to 90 percent cacao chocolate, finely chopped

1 tablespoon ghee or coconut oil

1. Preheat the oven to 200°F (for keeping finished pancakes warm).

2. In a large bowl, whisk together the eggs, water, and almond extract.

3. Add the coconut flour, tapioca starch, arrowroot starch, monk-fruit sweetener, baking powder, baking soda, and salt.

4. Mix until you have a smooth batter. Add the finely chopped chocolate and blend together.

5. Heat your griddle or ceramic nonstick pan to medium heat level, and put the ghee or coconut oil into the skillet or pan.

6. Use a little less than a quarter of a cup of batter to form 3-inch pancakes.

7. Once bubbles appear, flip pancakes and cook for an additional 2 to 3 minutes, or until golden brown.

8. Serve right out of the pan, or transfer to oven to keep warm. If you prefer to serve later or to freeze, you can put them in toaster oven to warm them up. (Let frozen pancakes defrost first for about an hour before toasting.)

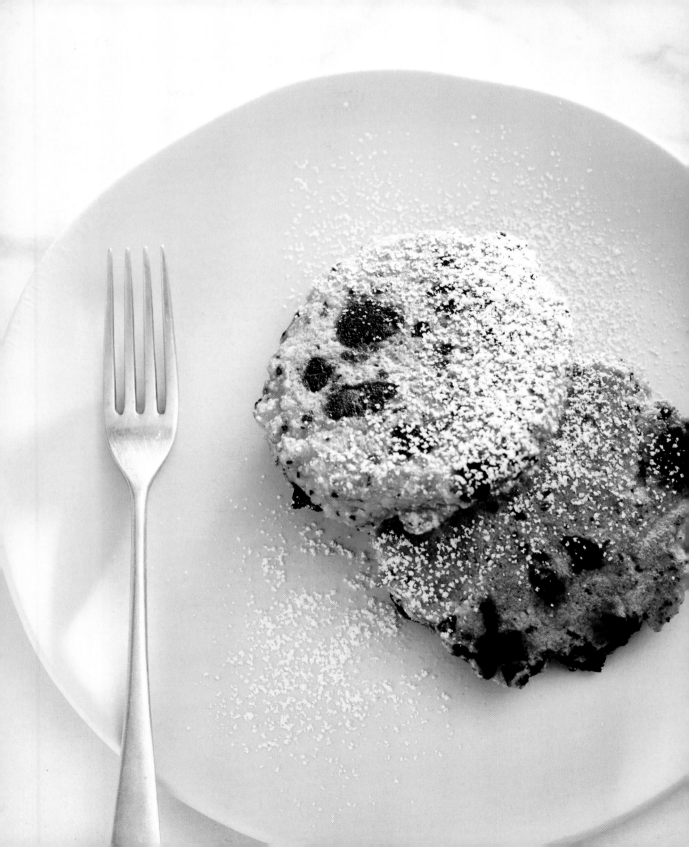

Broccoli Cheddar Quiche

This quiche is simple to whip up and makes a great plan-ahead breakfast when you have overnight visitors. I often prep my ingredients (and even bake the crust) the night before, so all I have to do is pop the quiche in the oven when my guests are waking up and voilà, a hot, satisfying breakfast appears effortless!

SERVES 8

FOR THE CRUST (or see Plant Paradox Piecrust, page 238)

1¼ cups coconut flour

½ cup toasted macadamia nuts, finely chopped

1 cup coconut oil

1 omega-3 or pastured egg or VeganEgg

FOR THE FILLING

2 cups broccoli florets, cut into small pieces

5 omega-3 or pastured eggs or VeganEggs

⅔ cup unsweetened coconut cream

¼ teaspoon nutmeg

1 teaspoon iodized sea salt

1 cup shredded goat's milk cheddar cheese or ½ cup nutritional yeast

1. Preheat the oven to 400°F. Spray an 8-inch pie tin with olive oil.

2. First, make the crust: pulse the coconut flour, macadamia nuts, coconut oil, and egg in a food processor until the mixture begins to come together. If too dry, add water 1 teaspoon at a time until the mixture becomes cohesive. The mixture will be a little crumbly, similar to a graham cracker crust.

3. Remove the dough from the food processor; press together in plastic wrap and refrigerate for 1 hour.

4. Press the dough into the pie tin using your fingertips, then bake for 10 minutes. Set aside and cool. Reduce oven temperature to 350°F.

5. Steam the broccoli for 2 to 3 minutes, then drain and set aside.

6. Combine the eggs, coconut cream, nutmeg, and salt, and mix well.

7. Place the crust on a sheet tray in case it overflows during baking.

8. Sprinkle cheddar cheese or nutritional yeast along the bottom of the crust, then add the broccoli.

9. Pour egg mixture over the top, and bake at 350°F for 35 to 40 minutes. Allow to cool for a few minutes before serving.

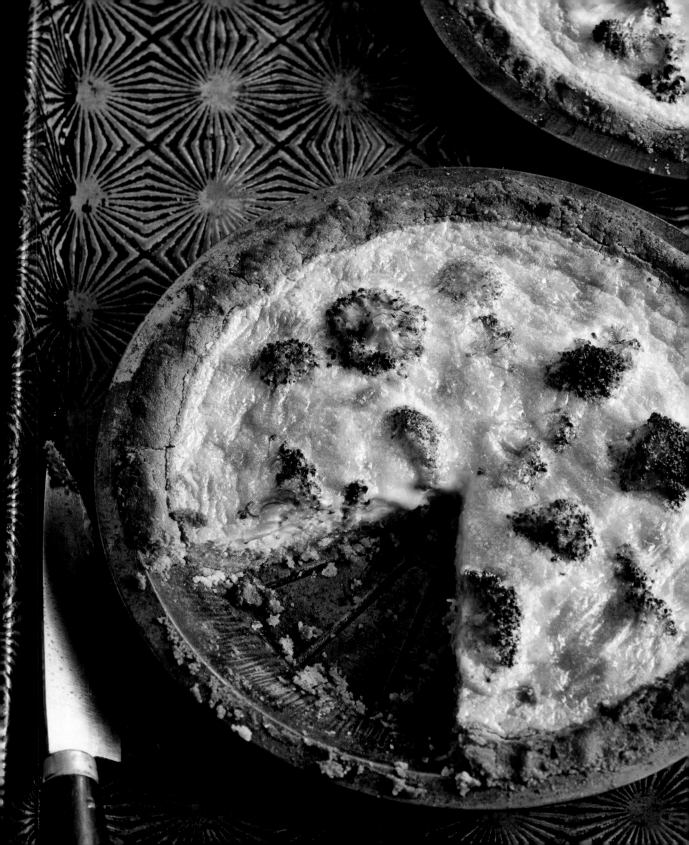

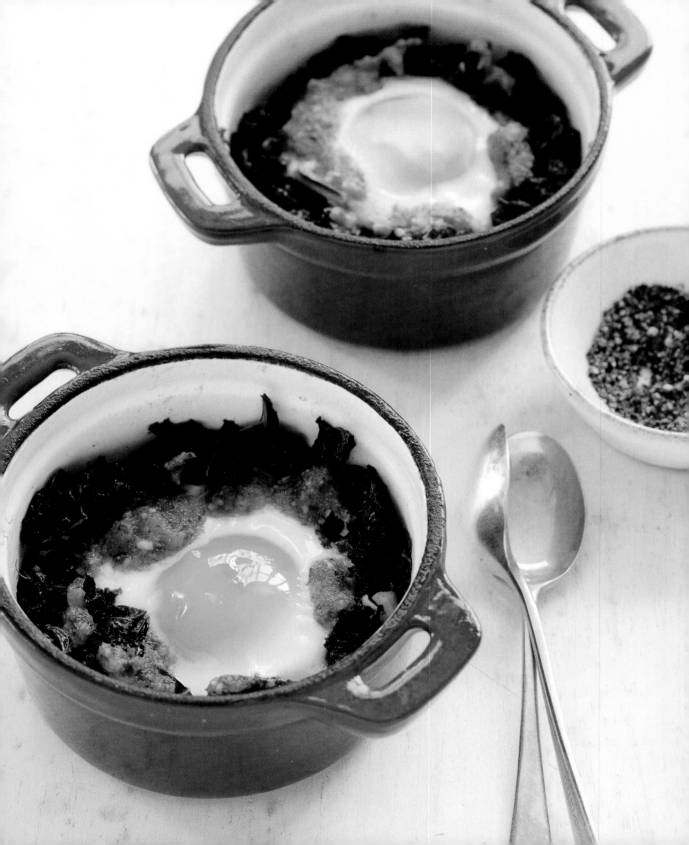

Pesto-Baked Eggs

This is one of my favorite brunch dishes because it's a great way to get greens (and olive oil) into your diet at the first meal of the day! Don't be alarmed if the pesto browns a bit—it'll still taste delicious.

SERVES 4

5 teaspoons extra-virgin olive oil

2 cups thinly sliced kale or Swiss chard

2 cloves garlic, minced

½ teaspoon iodized sea salt

4 omega-3 or pastured eggs or VeganEggs

4 tablespoons Classic Basil Pesto (page 258)

1. Preheat the oven to 350°F. Pour 1 teaspoon of olive oil into each of four 6- to 8-ounce ramekins.

2. In a large sauté pan, heat the remaining teaspoon of oil. Add kale or chard, garlic, and sea salt, and cook until kale is wilted and garlic is tender, about 3 minutes.

3. Divide garlic between ramekins, then crack 1 egg into each.

4. Top with pesto and bake 10 to 15 minutes, or until egg is set.

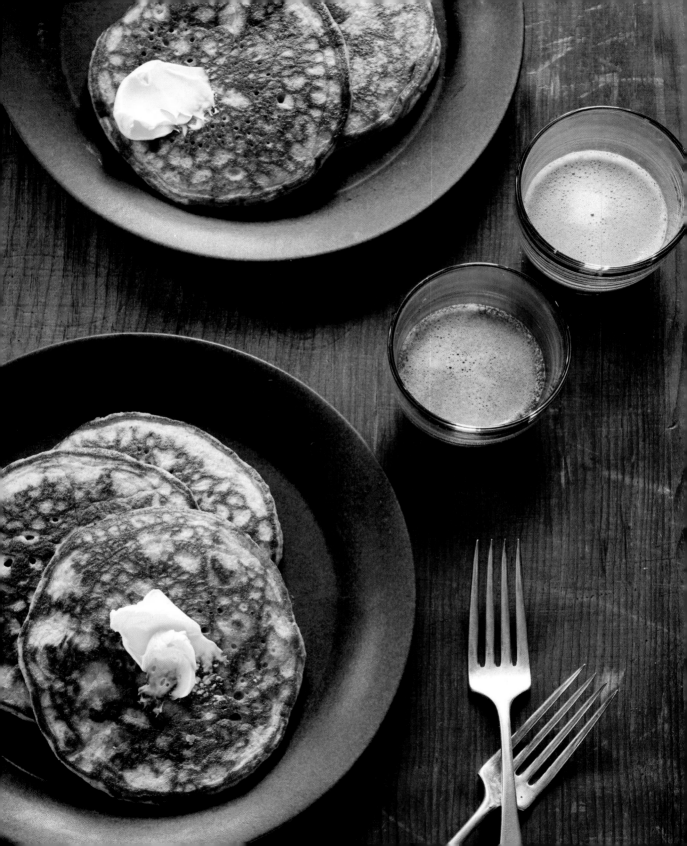

"Pumpkin" Spice Sweet Potato Pancakes

If you enjoy the pumpkin-spice craze but want to avoid the lectin-rich pumpkin that often accompanies it, these sweet potato pancakes hit the spot. They make for a special treat around the holidays, but you could serve them—for breakfast or dessert, with a little coconut cream—any time of year!

SERVES 1 TO 2

1 small sweet potato, baked, peeled, and mashed (approximately ½ cup)

4 to 5 drops stevia

2 teaspoons unsweetened coconut milk

2 omega-3 or pastured eggs or VeganEggs

½ teaspoon aluminum-free baking powder

3 tablespoons blanched almond flour

¼ teaspoon cinnamon

¼ teaspoon ground nutmeg

⅛ teaspoon ground cloves

¼ teaspoon ground ginger

Zest of 1 orange

French or Italian grass-fed butter (such as Trader Joe's Cultured French Butter, President, or Beurre D'Insigny), ghee, or avocado oil for cooking and serving

1. Whisk together the sweet potato, stevia, coconut milk, and eggs until well combined.

2. Add the baking powder, almond flour, spices, and orange zest to the mix.

3. Heat a skillet over medium-high heat and add butter. When it is melted, pour one-third of a cup of pancake batter into skillet and cook for 3 to 4 minutes. Flip with a spatula and cook an additional 3 to 4 minutes, or until golden brown.

4. Repeat with remaining batter and serve.

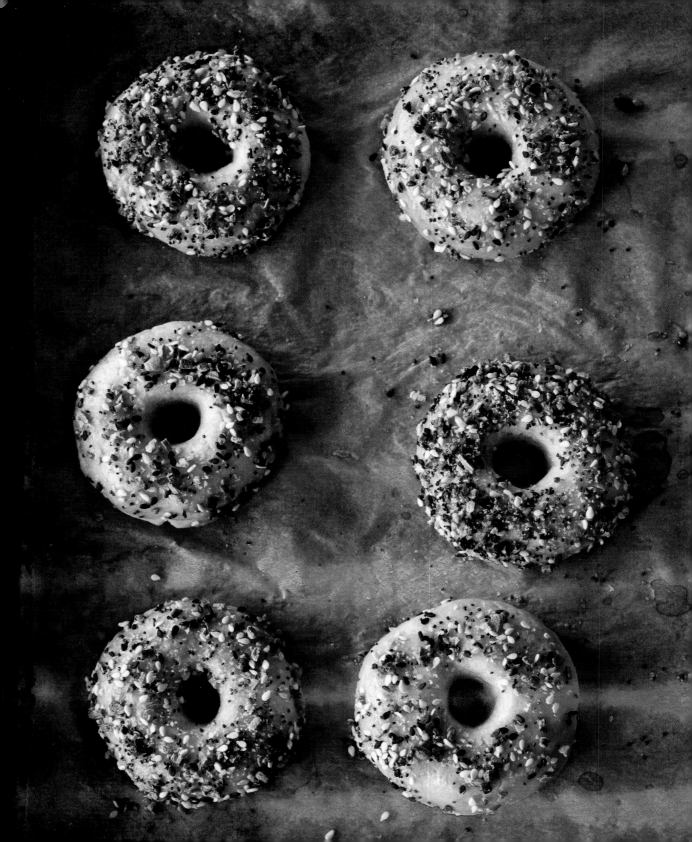

Plant Paradox Mini-Bagels

These lectin-free bagels don't taste like the big, doughy, glutinous bagels you might be used to, but I've actually come to prefer the flavor and texture of these more delicate mini-bagels. Try topping them with some smoked salmon and a smear of organic, full-fat cream cheese, grass-fed butter, or a scrambled, pastured egg and a few slices of avocado for a complete meal.

MAKES 11 TO 12 SMALL BAGELS

2 teaspoons plus ¼ teaspoon iodized sea salt

3 cups blanched almond flour

1 cup tapioca starch (plus additional for boiled water)

2 teaspoon baking powder

2 tablespoons monk-fruit sweetener (use a spice grinder to make into powder) or 1 packet stevia

2 tablespoons champagne or white wine vinegar

1 omega-3 or pastured egg or VeganEgg

Toppings of choice

1. Preheat the oven to 400°F. Place parchment paper on a baking sheet and set aside.

2. Fill a 10-inch pot with about 5 inches of water and add the quarter teaspoon of salt. Slowly bring the water to a boil.

3. In a medium bowl, combine the almond flour, tapioca starch, the remaining salt, baking powder, and monk-fruit powder.

4. Before water is at a full boil, remove half a cup and set aside.

5. Add the half cup of warm water and the vinegar to the dry mix. If the dough is too sticky, sprinkle lightly with more tapioca starch. If it's too dry, add a little more water.

6. Divide the dough into small balls on the baking sheet. You should have about 11 to 12 mini-bagels.

7. Flatten each ball with your hand and mold into the shape of a bagel. Use a utensil or your finger to make a small hole in the center of each. Each finished bagel should be about two and a quarter inches in diameter.

8. In groups of 3 or 4, carefully place the bagels in the boiling water.

(continued)

9. Using a strainer, remove them from the water once they float to the top, or after about 1 minute. Place the bagels back onto the baking sheet.

10. After boiling, bake the bagels for 10 minutes. While they are baking, put the egg in a small bowl and whisk.

11. Remove the bagels from the oven and brush each one with the beaten egg, adding your desired toppings before moving on to the next bagel. (This prevents the egg from drying before the toppings adhere.)

12. Return bagels to oven and bake for an additional 10 minutes. Increase temperature to 425°F. and bake for another 5 to 10 minutes, or until the bottoms of the bagels are just golden.

SUGGESTED TOPPINGS: *Trader Joe's "Everything But the Bagel"* (*toasted onion flakes, poppy seeds, toasted and black sesame seeds*), *caraway seeds, herbs de Provence, or rosemary and sea salt*

Spanish-Ish Omelet

When I first visited Spain I was blown away by the quality of the food. I was especially taken with the tortilla Española—the classic Spanish omelet made from thinly sliced potatoes, plenty of onions, and farm-fresh eggs. My lectin-free version, which uses sweet potatoes, is just as satisfying. Enjoy for breakfast or add a simple green salad to make a tasty, one-pan dinner.

SERVES 9

6 omega-3 or pastured eggs or VeganEggs

¼ cup minced parsley

½ teaspoon iodized sea salt

½ teaspoon paprika

½ teaspoon ground black pepper

2 tablespoons extra-virgin olive oil

1 cup thinly sliced sweet potatoes

1 sweet onion (such as Vidalia or Maui), thinly sliced

2 cups baby spinach

1. Preheat the oven to 425°F. Whisk the eggs, parsley, sea salt, paprika, and pepper in a large bowl, then set aside.

2. Heat 1 tablespoon of the olive oil in a medium oven-safe skillet over medium heat and add the sweet potatoes and onions.

3. Cook, stirring occasionally, until the sweet potatoes are tender and the onions are translucent, 8 to 10 minutes.

4. Add the spinach to the potato mixture and cook until wilted, an additional 2 minutes.

5. Drain the liquid from the potato mixture, then return to the heat along with the remaining olive oil.

6. Pour the eggs over the sweet potato mixture and cook, stirring occasionally, until eggs begin to set, 3 to 5 minutes.

7. Transfer skillet to oven and cook for an additional 5 to 7 minutes, until set.

8. Slice and serve.

"Bacon"-and-Egg Breakfast Salad

Salad for breakfast? Absolutely! It may not seem like an obvious choice, but when you take traditional breakfast ingredients, add greens, and top it all off with a tangy dressing, you have a salad that's sure to become a new favorite. As a Californian, I find this filling and refreshing dish especially great for those summer mornings where it's 80 degrees before 7:00 A.M.

SERVES 2

Juice of 1 lemon

¼ cup red wine vinegar

½ cup extra-virgin olive oil

½ teaspoon Dijon mustard

2 cups baby spinach

2 cups shredded kale, stems removed

2 hard-boiled eggs, chopped

3 ounces prosciutto, finely chopped, or vegan bacon pieces

½ cup broccoli slaw (shredded broccoli stalks sold in bags in the produce section)

½ avocado, diced

¼ cup unsweetened dried cranberries

1. In a large bowl, whisk together the lemon juice, red wine vinegar, olive oil, and mustard.

2. Add the spinach and kale to the bowl and toss to combine.

3. Top with eggs, prosciutto or vegan bacon, broccoli slaw, avocado, and dried cranberries. Enjoy immediately.

Omelet, Classic and Variations

The beauty of the classic omelet is its versatility—not only is it great at breakfast, but it's one of those foods that can really work at any time of day. In fact, most of the chefs I know consider an omelet a go-to dinner after a long, exhausting evening shift.

Once you know how to prepare a classic plain omelet, the possibilities are endless. Below, I've included instructions for a few of my favorite variations, as well as a quick tutorial on how to cook a perfect omelet.

For my vegan friends, check out VeganEgg—a plant-based egg substitute that cooks up just like a regular egg.

SERVES 1

2 omega-3 or pastured eggs or VeganEggs

Pinch of iodized sea salt

1 tablespoon French or Italian grass-fed butter (such as Trader Joe's Cultured French Butter, President, or Beurre D'Insigny) or extra-virgin olive oil

1. Crack the eggs into a small mixing bowl and add salt. Whisk gently with a fork until well beaten.

2. Heat an 8-inch skillet over medium heat; add the butter or olive oil.

3. When the butter, if using, is melted, slowly pour the egg mixture into the pan, tilting the pan to spread egg mixture evenly. Cook for 4 to 5 minutes, periodically pulling back a small section of the edge to let more uncooked egg come in contact with the pan surface, until the mixture holds together. (It will still be slightly wet in the middle—the center continues to cook after you fold it.)

4. Tilt the pan to one side and use a spatula to fold a third of the omelet into the middle (like folding a piece of paper to fit in an envelope.)

5. Holding the pan above a serving plate, tip the pan so the omelet rolls off, folding the remaining third of the omelet underneath.

6. Serve as is, or with salad.

(continued)

Herb

To make an herb omelet, add 1 to 2 tablespoons of fresh herbs to the egg mixture before cooking. I suggest minced parsley, thyme, and dill. If desired, add a tablespoon of grated Parmesan cheese to the mixture as well.

Mushroom

Sauté half a cup of diced mushrooms with 1 tablespoon olive oil or butter and one-half teaspoon fresh thyme leaves. Set filling aside. When folding the omelet (step 4), add mushroom mixture to the center of the omelet and fold eggs around it.

Green Eggs and Ham

Whisk 1 tablespoon of Classic Basil Pesto (page 258) into your eggs before cooking, then cook according to instructions for classic omelet. When folding, add 1 slice of prosciutto to the eggs.

Spinach

Sauté 1 cup of baby spinach in 1 tablespoon of extra-virgin olive oil over medium-high heat. When spinach has wilted, add a pinch of iodized sea salt, a tiny pinch of nutmeg, and a tablespoon of grated Parmesan. Set filling aside, then fold into eggs at step 4, before serving.

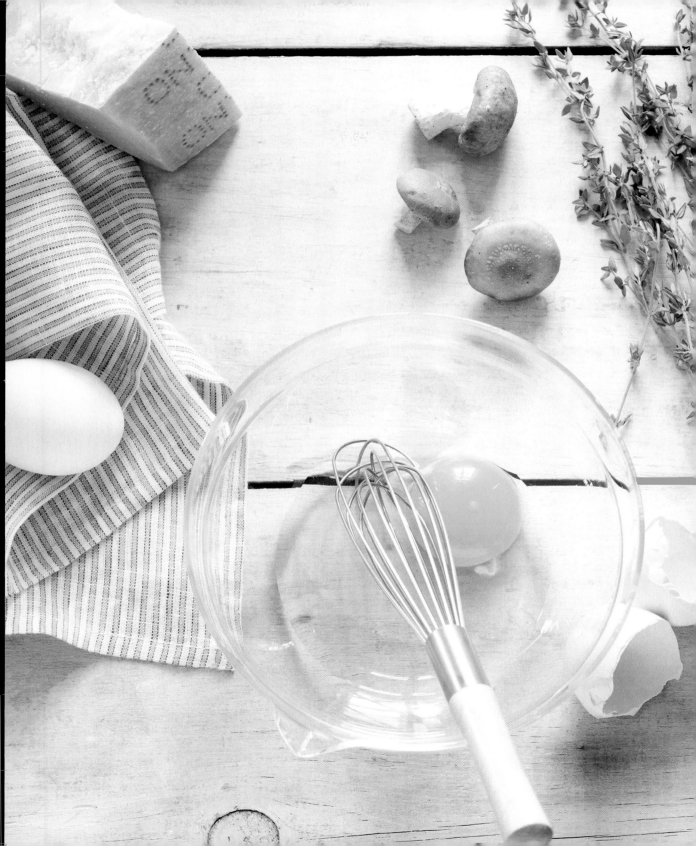

Walnut Bread

Think of this bread as a gut-friendly twist on rye bread—a little sweet, a little sour, a bit dense, and great for sandwiches, lightly buttered, or topped with organic, full-fat cream cheese. If you prefer a bread with a lighter texture, you can skip the hazelnut flour and substitute 2 cups of almond flour.

MAKES 1 LOAF

4 tablespoons avocado or coconut oil, melted, plus additional for greasing the pan

1½ cup blanched almond flour

½ cup hazelnut flour (available at Trader Joe's, or grind your own)

6 tablespoons arrowroot starch

4 tablespoons finely ground flaxseeds

1 cup diced walnuts

2 tablespoons tapioca starch

½ teaspoon iodized sea salt

¾ teaspoon baking soda

4 large omega-3 or pastured eggs or VeganEggs

½ cup plain full-fat coconut milk

2 tablespoons yacón syrup

1½ teaspoons red wine vinegar

1. Preheat the oven to 350°F. Generously grease an 8½ × 4½-inch glass or metal loaf pan with avocado or coconut oil (or you can line it with parchment).

2. Whisk together the almond flour, hazelnut flour, arrowroot starch, flaxseeds, walnuts, tapioca starch, salt, and baking soda in a large bowl.

3. In a smaller bowl, combine the avocado or coconut oil, eggs, coconut milk, yacón syrup, and vinegar.

4. Add the wet ingredients to the dry all at once and stir until combined, being careful not to over-mix (too much mixing makes the bread tough).

5. Immediately pour the batter into the prepared pan and bake until a toothpick inserted into the center comes out clean, about 40 to 45 minutes.

6. Cool on a wire rack before slicing and serving, and store any leftovers wrapped in the fridge for up to 5 days.

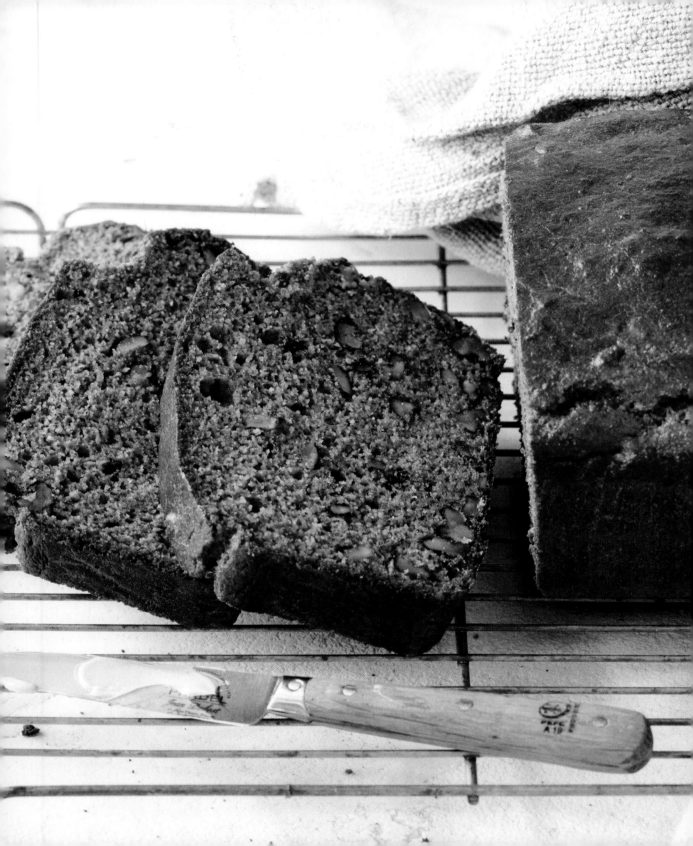

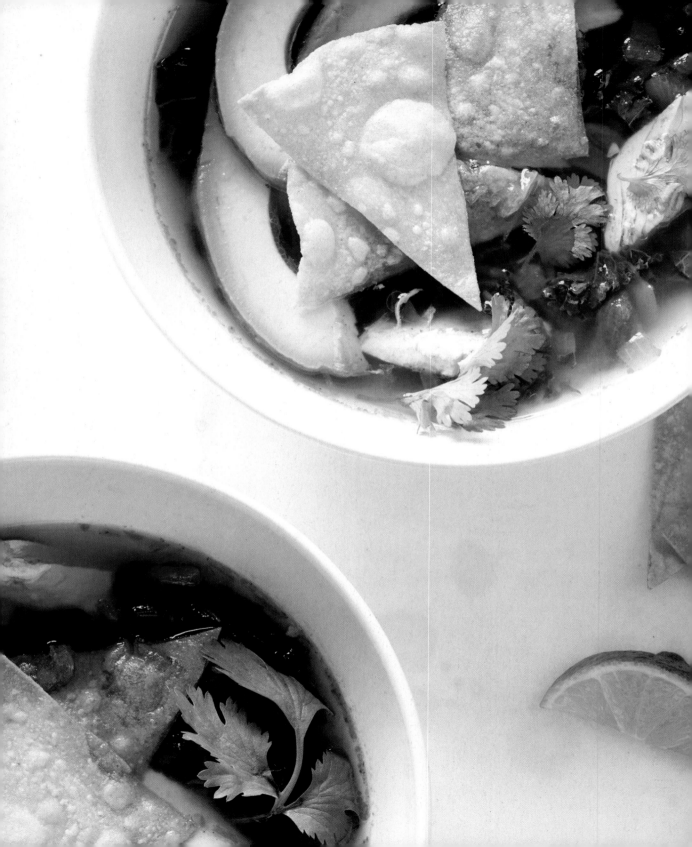

chapter seven

_____

Soups and Stews

_____

Chicken and Vegetable (Miracle) Rice Soup

Chicken and rice is a classic soup combination, perfect when you're feeling under the weather or anytime you need a pick-me-up. My version delivers the same healing properties, minus the lectins! If you're making a larger batch to freeze, leave out the Miracle Rice and add it as you reheat to prevent it from getting mushy.

SERVES 4

¼ cup extra-virgin olive oil

1 onion, diced

3 celery stalks, diced

2 cloves garlic, minced

2 cups mushrooms, diced

1 teaspoon dried sage

1 teaspoon fresh thyme

½ teaspoon fresh rosemary

½ teaspoon black pepper

Zest of 1 lemon

Juice of 1 lemon

1 teaspoon iodized sea salt

1 cup diced cooked pasture-raised chicken or Quorn crumbles

4 cups Bone Broth (page 257) or organic, low-sodium chicken or vegetable broth

2 packages Miracle Rice

1. In a large soup pot, heat the olive oil over medium-high heat. Add the onion and celery, and cook until tender and translucent, 5 or 6 minutes.

2. Add the garlic and mushrooms, along with sage, thyme, rosemary, pepper, lemon zest, lemon juice, and salt, and cook, stirring regularly, until tender, approximately 3 to 5 minutes.

3. Add chicken (or Quorn) and broth, then reduce heat to low and simmer for 15 to 20 minutes. Add Miracle Rice and cook until heated through, 1 to 2 minutes, before serving.

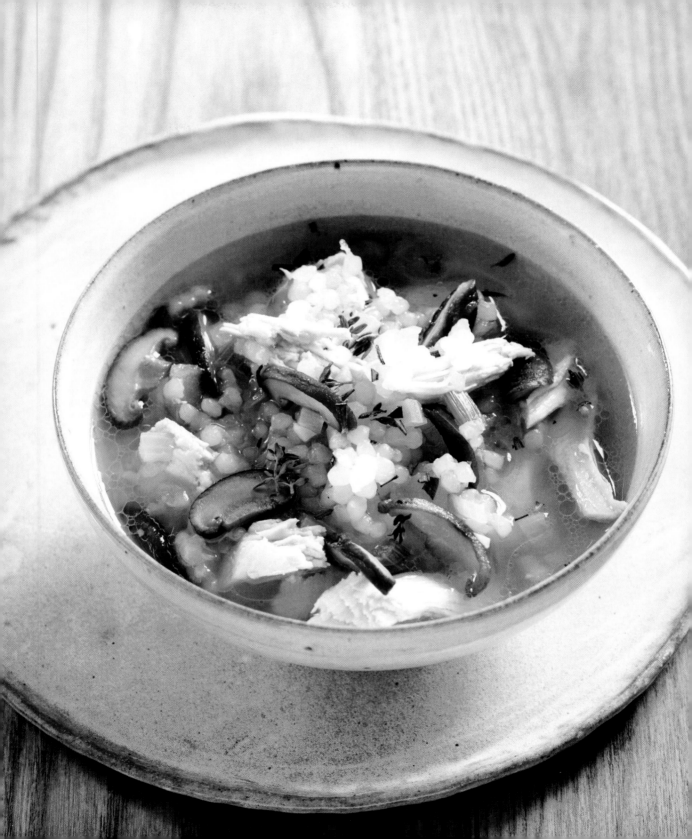

Creamy Sweet Potato Soup

I used to order butternut squash or pumpkin soup whenever I saw it on a restaurant menu—I love the flavor of squash—but for a long time I didn't know that squash was less fond of me. If you enjoy these flavors as much as I do, this sweet-savory, velvety smooth soup is going to become a go-to in your recipe arsenal.

SERVES 4 TO 6

2 tablespoons extra-virgin olive oil

1 small onion, diced

3 celery stalks, diced

3 to 4 sweet potatoes (about 2 pounds), peeled and cut into 1-inch cubes

2 cloves garlic, chopped

1 to 2 teaspoons iodized sea salt

1 teaspoon freshly ground black pepper

1 teaspoon paprika

1 teaspoon fresh thyme

½ teaspoon cinnamon

4 cups chicken stock or Vegetable Stock (page 265)

Parmesan cheese, to garnish (optional)

Extra fresh ground black pepper, to taste

1. Heat the olive oil over medium-high heat in a large soup pot. Add the onion and celery and sauté until tender and translucent.

2. Add the sweet potatoes, garlic, sea salt, pepper, paprika, thyme, and cinnamon, and sauté until the thyme is fragrant and the sweet potatoes begin to become tender at the edges.

3. Add the stock and reduce heat to low. Cover and simmer for 30 minutes, until sweet potatoes are falling apart.

4. Transfer the mixture to a high-speed blender (or use an immersion blender) and blend until smooth.

5. Serve garnished with cheese (if using) and black pepper.

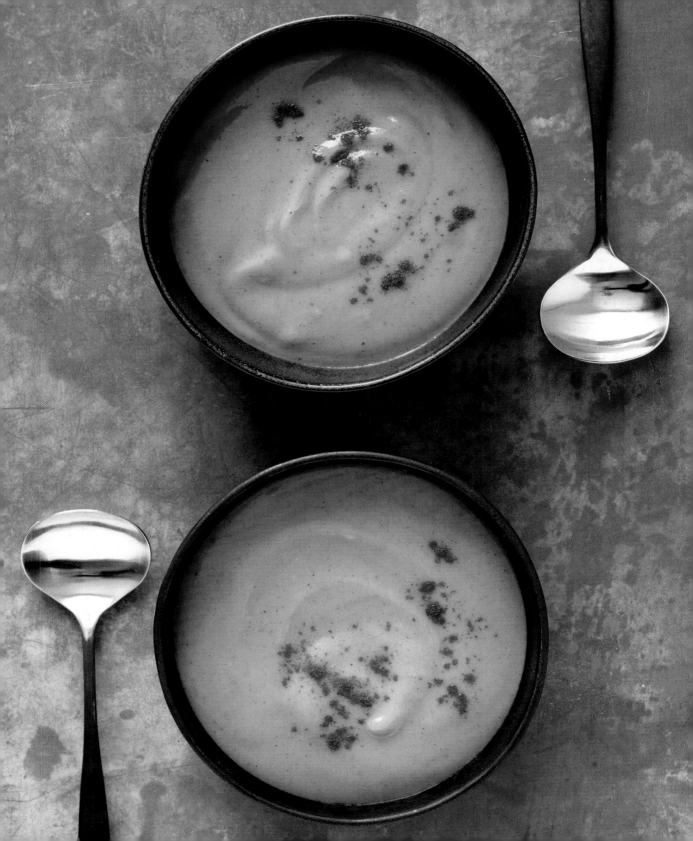

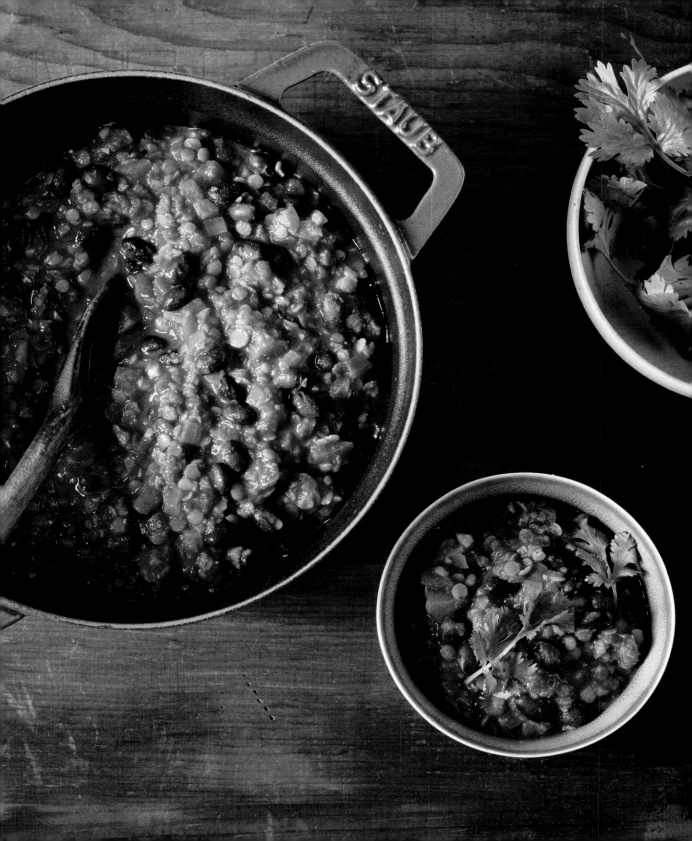

Dr. G's Bean Chili

Yes, your read that right: This is a bean-based chili. By pressure-cooking this chili, you reduce the lectin content, making it 100 percent doable on Phase 3 of the Plant Paradox program. And since it's made in a pressure cooker, it also comes together in a snap. No more simmering chili on the stove for hours!

SERVES 4

¼ cup olive oil

1 large onion, chopped

5 cloves garlic, minced

1 red bell pepper, peeled, seeded, and chopped

1 poblano pepper, peeled, seeded, and chopped

1 jalapeño pepper, peeled, seeded, and diced

1 cup dried red beans, picked over, rinsed, and soaked 24–48 hours in 2 changes of water

1 cup dried black beans, picked over, rinsed, and soaked in 2 changes of water

1 cup dried lentils, picked over, and soaked in 2 changes of water

5 cups peeled, seeded, and minced tomatoes (about 7 tomatoes)

3 cups water or vegetable broth

2 tablespoons chili powder

1 tablespoon chipotle puree (optional, but recommended)

1 tablespoon ground cumin

1 teaspoon iodized sea salt, more to taste

½ cup shredded goat's milk cheddar, to serve (optional)

1 cup diced cilantro, to serve (optional)

1. In a large pot (or in a pressure cooker on sauté setting), heat the olive oil over medium-high heat.

2. Sauté the onions, garlic, and peppers until very fragrant, about 5 to 7 minutes, then transfer to the pressure cooker.

3. Add the beans, lentils, tomatoes, broth or water, spices, including chipotle puree if desired, and salt and stir well to combine.

4. Cook on high pressure for about 10 minutes, according to the instructions on your pressure cooker.

5. Let pressure cooker depressurize, then remove from heat, stir, and serve. Garnish with cheddar or cilantro if desired.

Leek and Cauliflower Soup

Leek and potato soup is one of those unusual dishes that's good hot, at room temperature, or even chilled. This simple variation on the classic is just as versatile. It never ceases to amaze me how well cauliflower works in place of potatoes in most dishes.

SERVES 4 TO 6

3 tablespoons extra-virgin olive oil

1 pound leeks, cleaned and chopped

2 celery stalks, diced

3 cloves garlic, minced

1 large head of cauliflower, cut into 2-inch florets

½ teaspoon fresh nutmeg

1 teaspoon fine iodized sea salt, or more, to taste

2 teaspoons coarse black pepper

2 quarts salt-free chicken stock or Vegetable Stock (page 265)

¼ cup grated Parmesan (optional, but delicious)

1 bay leaf

Finely chopped chives or thyme, to garnish

1. Heat the olive oil over medium-high heat in a large soup pot. Add the leeks, celery, garlic, and cauliflower, along with the nutmeg, salt, and pepper, and sauté over medium, stirring regularly until leeks begin to wilt.

2. Add stock, Parmesan (if using), and bay leaf, and cook, covered, for 35 to 45 minutes, until cauliflower is very tender.

3. Remove bay leaf and blend using an immersion stick blender, or transfer into a regular blender and blend until smooth (work in batches so as to not overfill the blender).

4. Once pureed, return the soup to the heat and cook an additional 10 to 15 minutes.

5. Serve garnished with chopped herbs and more Parmesan, if desired.

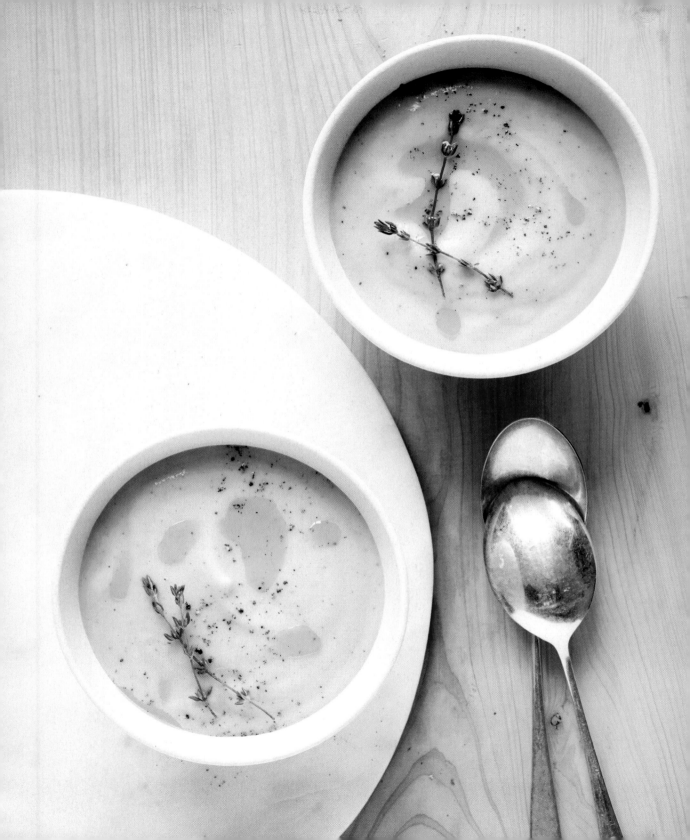

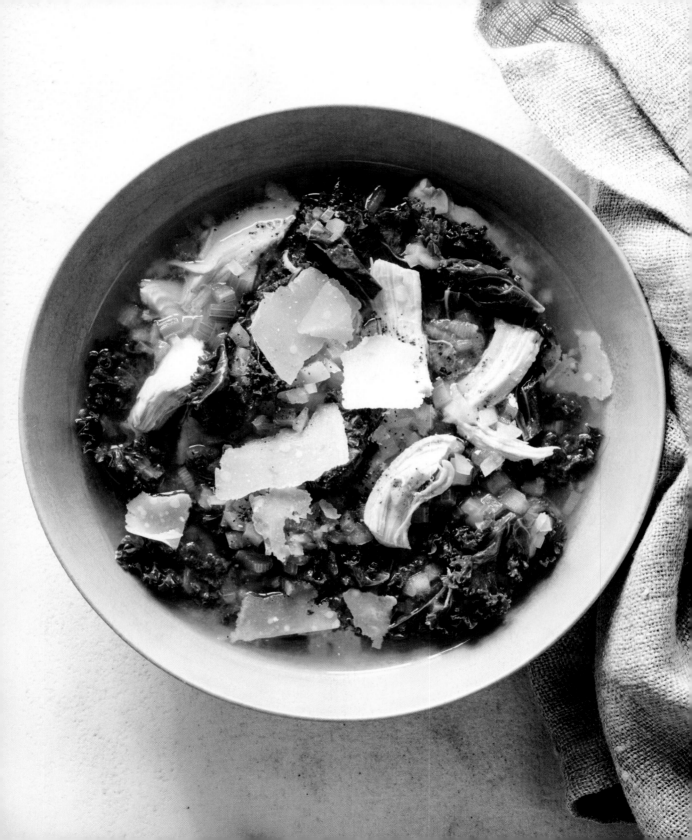

Lemon, Kale, and Chicken Soup

I first came up with this recipe to share with the readers of my blog, and it's quickly become not only a fan favorite, but a meal I keep in my weekly rotation. I make a big batch and freeze it in pint jars for easy single-serving meals.

SERVES 4 TO 6

3 tablespoons extra-virgin olive oil

1 medium onion, finely diced

4 cloves garlic, minced

2 celery stalks, minced

Freshly ground black pepper, to taste

Iodized sea salt, to taste

1 cup cooked pastured chicken (white or dark meat—perfect for using up whatever leftover chicken you have on hand), cubed or shredded, or 1 cup Quorn crumbles

½ teaspoon Dijon mustard

2 bunches kale, cut into 1-inch pieces

Zest of 1 lemon

5 cups Chicken Bone Broth (page 257) or Vegetable Stock (page 265)

1 teaspoon balsamic vinegar

2 tablespoons fresh lemon juice

Freshly grated Parmigiano Reggiano, for serving (optional)

1. Heat the olive oil over medium heat in a large soup pot. Add the onion, garlic, and celery, along with the black pepper and a *tiny* pinch of the sea salt. Sauté until onions and celery are very tender.

2. Add the chicken or Quorn, mustard, kale, and lemon zest, and sauté for an additional 5 minutes.

3. Add the stock, balsamic vinegar, and lemon juice, and reduce heat. Cook, covered, for 35 minutes.

4. Ladle into bowls and top with fresh black pepper and cheese, if desired.

"Cream" of Mushroom Soup

My family loves to serve cream of mushroom soup as a special holiday entrée, and this simple variation on the classic is just as decadent! It gets its creaminess from an unexpected source—cauliflower—with just a hint of coconut cream stirred in at the end.

SERVES 8

3 tablespoons extra-virgin olive oil

2 pounds mushrooms, finely diced

1 teaspoon fresh thyme

Zest of 1 lemon

1 onion, diced

2 cloves garlic, minced

2 celery stalks, diced

1 large head cauliflower, outer leaves removed, coarsely chopped

1½ teaspoons iodized sea salt

½ teaspoon black pepper

½ teaspoon onion powder

1 teaspoon Dijon mustard

4 cups Bone Broth (page 257) or organic, low-sodium chicken or vegetable broth

1 cup unsweetened coconut cream

1. In a large soup pot, heat 2 tablespoons of the olive oil over medium heat. Add the mushrooms and cook until golden brown and tender, then add the thyme and lemon and cook for an additional 2 minutes, until very fragrant.

2. Set half the mushrooms aside, leaving the rest in the pot. Add the remaining olive oil, along with the onion, garlic, and celery, and cook until onion and celery are tender.

3. Add the cauliflower to the pot, along with the salt, pepper, onion powder, and mustard.

4. Sauté until fragrant, then add the broth. Cook until cauliflower is tender, 5 to 7 minutes, then transfer to a blender to puree.

5. When soup is smooth, add the reserved mushrooms and the coconut cream. Stir to combine and serve.

Mushroom Coconut Curry

I love traditional Thai curries for their richness and their depth of flavor. This creamy, aromatic vegetable curry is delicious over cauliflower rice or on its own. And strange as it may sound, it pairs really well with a nice glass of a crisp, dry sparkling wine.

SERVES 8

1 tablespoon coconut oil

1 small white onion, diced

2 cloves garlic, pressed or minced

1 tablespoon minced fresh ginger

2 cups broccoli slaw (the packaged, shredded broccoli stalks available in the produce section of most grocery stores)

2 cups sliced brown mushrooms

2 tablespoons Thai red curry paste

1 14-ounce can unsweetened coconut milk

½ cup water or broth

1½ cups packed thinly sliced kale

5 to 6 drops stevia

1 tablespoon fish sauce or coconut aminos

Juice of 1 lime

1 small handful basil or cilantro, chopped

1. Heat the oil over medium-high heat in a large soup pot. Add the onion, and cook until translucent, then add the garlic and ginger.

2. When the garlic and ginger are fragrant, add the broccoli slaw and mushrooms and cook over medium-high heat until tender, about 4 to 6 minutes.

3. Add the curry paste, and stir until well incorporated. Cook 1 to 2 minutes, until very fragrant.

4. Add the coconut milk and water or broth, as well as the kale, stevia, and fish sauce and reduce heat to low. Simmer for 20 minutes, then remove from heat. Add the lime juice, and basil or cilantro, and serve.

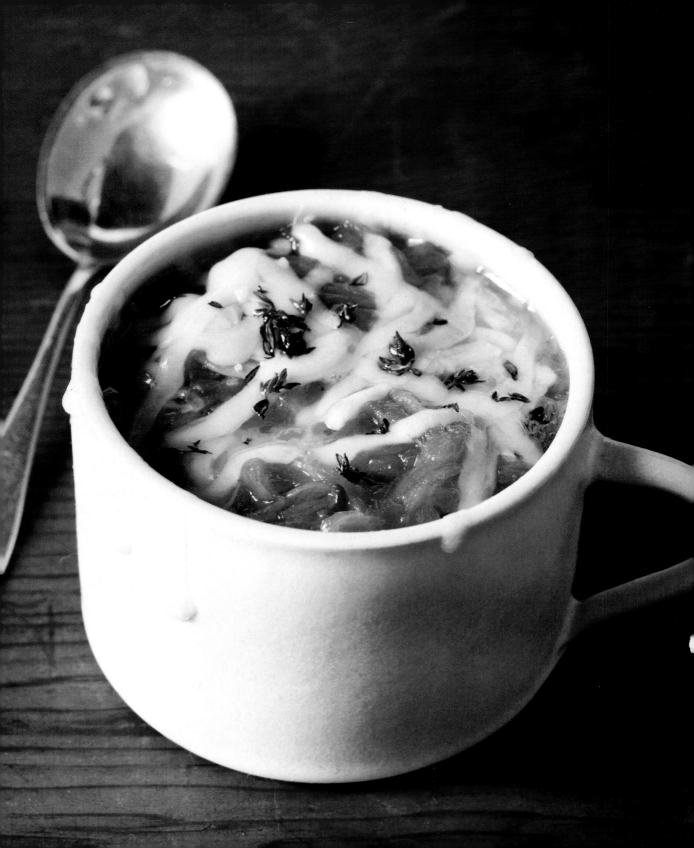

Not-Quite-French Onion Soup

Nothing beats a steaming hot bowl of French onion soup . . . but between the croutons, the beef broth, the gobs of cheese, and the added sugar (yes, really), it's not great for your gut. This vegetarian French onion soup has all the classic comfort, minus the lectins. To make it really special, try using homemade bone broth in place of the vegetable stock.

SERVES 6 TO 8

¼ cup extra-virgin olive oil

5 large sweet onions (like Maui or Vidalia), thinly sliced

2 tablespoons red wine vinegar

6 cloves garlic, thinly sliced

2 bay leaves

1 teaspoon chopped fresh thyme

½ teaspoon ground black pepper

6 cups Bone Broth (page 257) or Vegetable Stock (page 265) or water, or a combination of the three

Iodized sea salt, to taste

Grated Gruyère or Parmesan cheese, to taste, for serving

1. Heat the olive oil over low heat. Add the onions, and cook, stirring frequently, until the onions are dark brown and caramelized, about 15 minutes.

2. Add the vinegar and garlic, and reduce heat to low. Cook, stirring frequently, until garlic is fragrant, about 2 minutes.

3. Add bay leaves, thyme, pepper, and broth or stock, and cook, covered, for 15 to 20 minutes. Uncover and cook another 10 to 15 minutes before removing from the heat. Remove bay leaves and season with salt to taste.

4. Ladle soup into ramekins or small bowls and top with grated cheese. If the heat of the soup isn't enough to melt the cheese, pop the oven-safe bowls on a sheet pan and place under the broiler for 30 seconds to 1 minute.

Pressure Cooker Black Bean Soup with Avocado Salsa

This soup is delicious on its own, but becomes positively decadent when topped with a dollop of coconut yogurt or avocado salsa. I like to serve it with Cassava Chips for a meal that's even better than your favorite Mexican takeout.

SERVES 6 TO 8

FOR THE SOUP
¼ cup extra-virgin olive oil

1 large yellow onion, diced

1 tablespoon mild chili powder

1½ teaspoons whole cumin seeds

1½ teaspoons dried oregano

½ teaspoon paprika

1 teaspoon non-Dutched cocoa powder

7 cups mushroom broth or Bone Broth (page 257)

1 pound (2½ cups) dried black beans, picked over and rinsed in 2 changes of water

6 cloves garlic, minced

2 bay leaves

Iodized sea salt, to taste

Your favorite hot sauce, to taste

FOR THE AVOCADO SALSA
2 large ripe avocados, diced

⅓ cup chopped red onion

¼ cup chopped cilantro

½ cup pomegranate arils (in season, September through January)

1 jalapeño, peeled, seeded, and diced (optional)

1. In a 6-quart or larger pressure cooker, heat the oil over medium-high heat on the stove, or use the sauté function on a digital pressure cooker.

2. When oil is hot, add the onions, chili powder, cumin, oregano, paprika, and cocoa powder. Stir frequently until onions begin to soften, 2 to 3 minutes

3. Add the broth, beans, garlic, and bay leaves.

4. Lock the lid in place.

   For a stovetop pressure cooker: Over high heat, bring to high pressure. Reduce the heat just enough to maintain high pressure and cook for 30 minutes. Once time is up, allow the pressure to come down naturally, about 15 minutes. Remove the lid, tilting it away from you to allow the steam to escape.

   For an electric cooker: Cook on high pressure for 30 minutes, then release the pressure according to the manufacturer's instructions for your pressure cooker.

5. Stir well. Remove the bay leaves and add salt and hot sauce to taste.

6. Just before serving, prepare the avocado salsa by tossing

2 to 3 tablespoons freshly squeezed lime juice

1 cup coconut yogurt

Cassava Chips (page 36), for serving

the avocado, onion, cilantro, pomegranate arils, jalapeño, lime juice, and yogurt together in a bowl. Ladle the soup into bowls and top each portion with a large dollop of avocado salsa. Serve with chips, if desired.

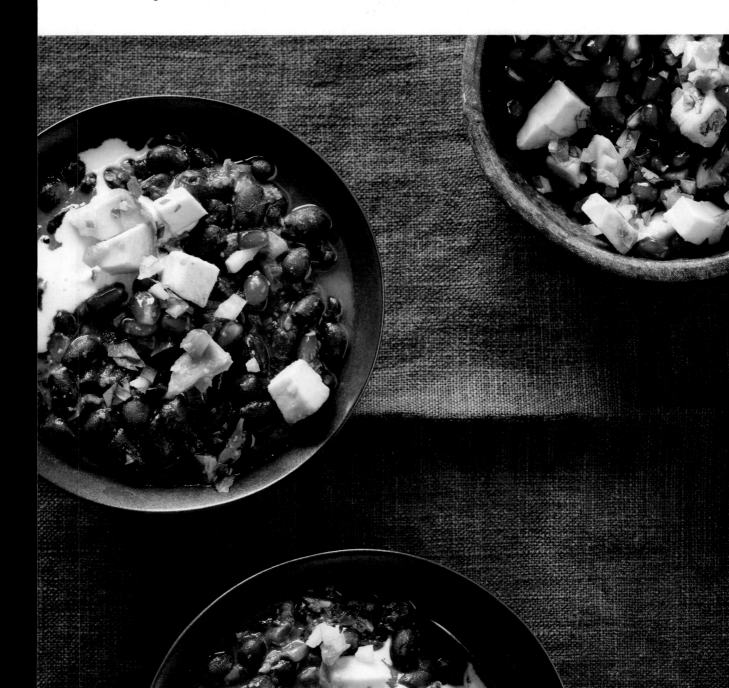

Beef and Mushroom Stew

This stew is stick-to-your-ribs kind of food—it makes for a warm, satisfying meal in cooler months. I like to serve it over mashed cauliflower or sweet potatoes for a hearty but not heavy meal.

SERVES 6 TO 8

1 pound pastured sirloin, cubed, or 16 ounces cubed tempeh

2 tablespoons cassava flour

¼ cup extra-virgin olive oil

1 large onion, diced

3 celery stalks, minced

3 cloves garlic, minced

1 pound mushrooms, sliced

1 teaspoon iodized sea salt

1 tablespoon fresh thyme leaves

1 cup red wine

2 cups Bone Broth (page 257) or vegetable broth

1 tablespoon red wine vinegar

1. In a bowl, toss the sirloin (or tempeh) with cassava flour until evenly coated.

2. Heat the olive oil in a large soup pot over medium heat.

3. Add the sirloin or tempeh, and sear on all sides until golden brown.

4. Add the onion, celery, garlic, and mushrooms, and cook, stirring regularly, until vegetables are tender and garlic is very fragrant (about 4 to 6 minutes).

5. Add the sea salt and thyme and sauté an additional minute, until fragrant.

6. Deglaze the pot with the wine, broth, and vinegar, making sure to scrape the bottom of the pan to lift off all the brown, cooked-on goodness.

7. Reduce heat to low and simmer for 45 minutes to 1 hour, adding water as needed, until beef is very tender.

8. Serve over mashed cauliflower or sweet potatoes.

Sweet Potato and Spinach Curry

This beautiful recipe comes courtesy of our GundryMD.com third-place recipe contest winner, Preethi Hulikeremath. We were hooked the second we tasted the rich yet perfectly balanced flavors, and we know you'll love this dish too—especially if you love Indian food. If you don't have all the spices Preethi recommends, try using two tablespoons of curry powder instead; the flavor won't be quite as complex, but it'll still be delicious.

SERVES 2 TO 4

3 to 4 teaspoons avocado oil

1⅓ teaspoon mustard seeds

⅓ teaspoon cumin seeds

1 green cardamom pod

3 whole cloves

3 minced garlic cloves

1 red onion, minced

1 medium sweet potato, peeled and diced

½ teaspoon turmeric

⅓ teaspoon cinnamon powder

1 teaspoon crushed black pepper

2 cups coconut milk or water

2 cups baby spinach

Iodized sea salt, to taste

1. Add 1 teaspoon of the avocado oil to a large stainless steel pan and heat over low heat, then add the mustard seeds and cumin seeds, and roast for about 20 seconds.

2. Add the cardamom and cloves, roast them for 1 minute, stirring frequently.

3. Remove from heat, and pulse in a spice grinder until powdery.

4. Add the remaining oil to the pan, along with the garlic and onion.

5. Sauté on a medium flame until garlic and onion are golden brown, about 2 to 4 minutes.

6. Add the sweet potato and sauté an additional 3 to 4 minutes, then add the turmeric, cinnamon, and black pepper, along with the powdered spices you roasted in steps 1 and 2.

7. Add the coconut milk or water as well as the spinach, and let cook for 15 to 20 minutes, until sweet potatoes are very tender.

8. Season with salt to taste, and serve.

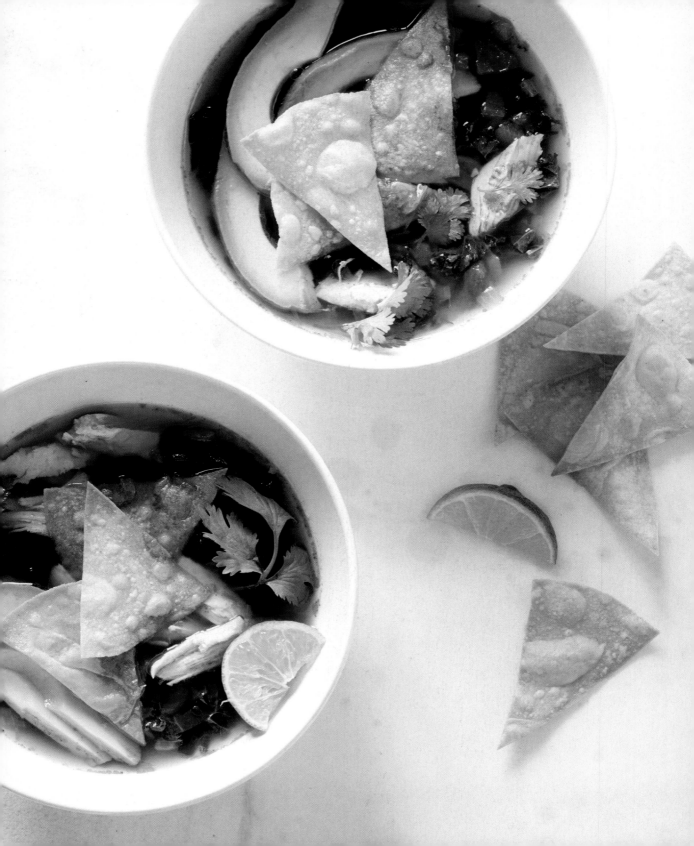

Tortilla Lime Soup

When I'm under the weather, I could drink the tangy broth that is the base of this soup with a straw—it's that good. I've included chicken in this recipe but you can omit it for a vegetarian version that is just as delicious.

SERVES 6

¼ cup extra-virgin olive oil

1 large yellow onion, diced

3 celery stalks, minced

2 garlic cloves, minced

1 teaspoon ground cumin

¾ teaspoon chili powder

1½ teaspoon salt, plus more to taste

6 cups vegetable broth

4 small tomatoes, peeled, seeded, and minced

2 cups thinly sliced kale, ribs removed

2 cups chopped cooked pastured chicken, skin removed (optional)

Juice of 4 limes

4 tablespoons chopped fresh cilantro

1 ½ ripe avocado, minced

1 cup Cassava Tortillas (and Chips) (page 36)

1. Heat the olive oil in a large soup pot over medium-high heat. Add the onion and celery and cook until tender and translucent, 3 to 5 minutes

2. Add the garlic, cumin, chili powder, and salt to the pot and cook, stirring frequently, until garlic is fragrant, about 2 minutes.

3. Add the vegetable broth and tomatoes and cook, covered, for 15 to 20 minutes.

4. Remove cover and stir in the kale, chicken (if using), and lime juice. Cook until kale is wilted, about 3 to 5 minutes, then add cilantro, avocado, and tortilla chips.

5. Remove from heat, taste and season if needed, and serve immediately.

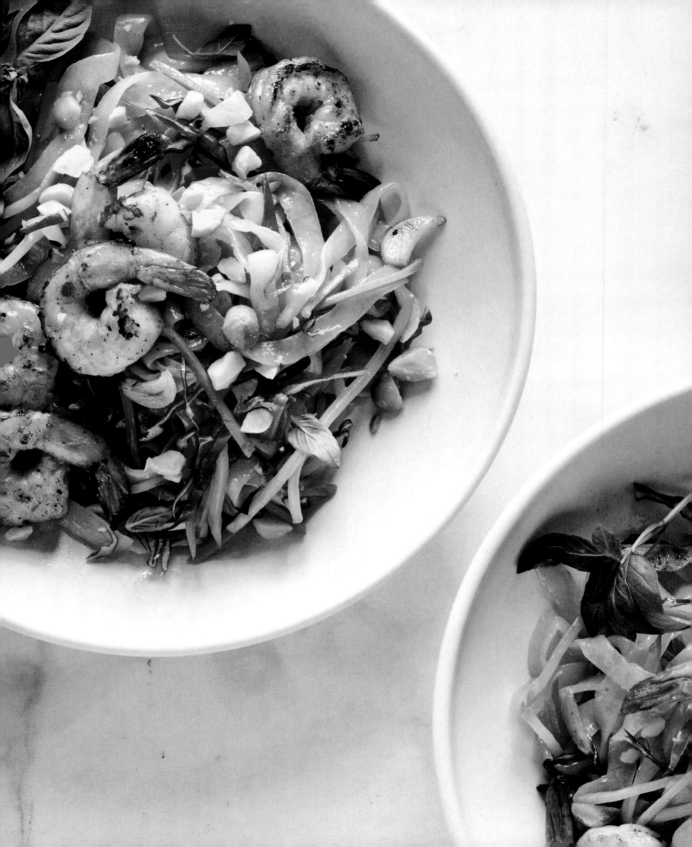

chapter eight

Noodles and Bowls

Banh Mi Bowl

If you've ever had a banh mi—the classic Vietnamese sandwich—you know it's addictive. And, of course, you know you probably shouldn't be eating that bread or that commercially farmed meat. But you *can* enjoy the tangy-sweet flavor of a classic banh mi—without the bun. Want it a little heartier? Serve over Miracle Rice or cauliflower rice instead of greens!

SERVES 1

DRESSING
¼ avocado

¼ cup cilantro

Juice of 1 lime

1 teaspoon garlic chili sauce or Sriracha

1 teaspoon sesame oil

1 teaspoon rice wine vinegar

BOWL
1 tablespoon toasted sesame oil

2 ounces pasture-raised chicken, diced, or ½ cup Quorn crumbles

½ teaspoon yacón syrup

½ teaspoon fish sauce or coconut aminos

½ teaspoon rice wine vinegar

2 cups mixed salad greens

¼ cup pickled daikon*

¼ cup pickled red onions*

¼ cup pickled carrots*

1 omega-3 or pastured egg, soft-boiled and peeled**

1. Make the dressing by pulsing all of the ingredients in a blender until smooth. Set aside.

2. In a sauté pan, heat the sesame oil over medium heat until warm and fragrant. Add the Quorn or chicken and sauté 3 to 4 minutes, stirring occasionally.

3. Add the yacón syrup, fish sauce or coconut aminos, and rice wine vinegar to the mix, and reduce heat to low. Continue cooking until the meat is cooked and mixture is nicely caramelized.

4. Toss the salad greens with the dressing, and place in your serving bowl.

5. Arrange meat, daikon, red onions, carrots, and the egg on top of the greens. Serve and enjoy!

Available in some Asian markets, or make your own Quick-Pickled Vegetables at home (page 208).

** *To soft-boil an egg, bring a pot of water to a rolling boil. Add the egg, and when water comes back to a boil, cook for 6 to 7 minutes. Transfer the egg to a bowl of ice water and peel it immediately.*

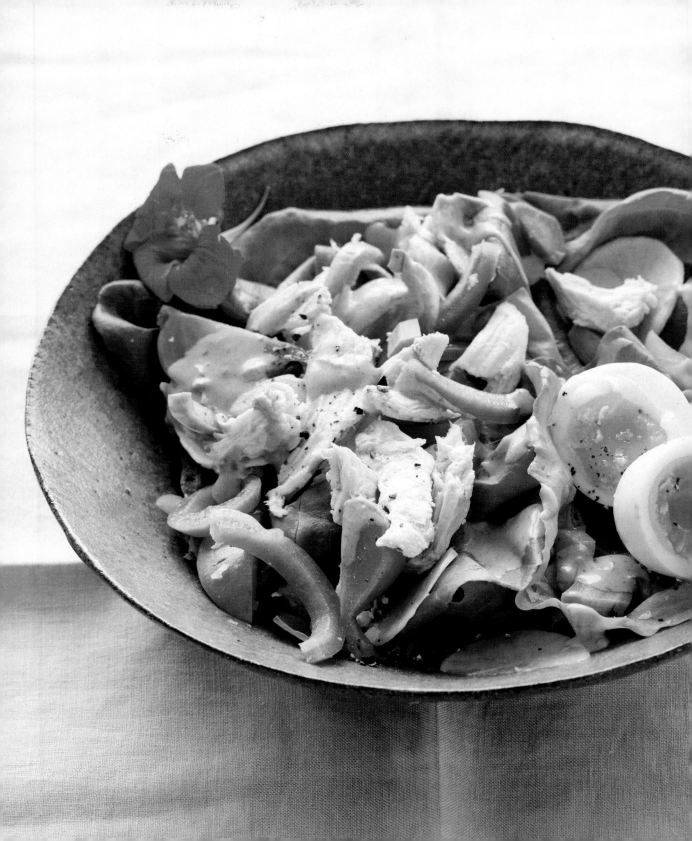

Burrito Bowl

Inspired by everyone's favorite fast-food chain burrito (I won't name names here, but you know who they are—it usually weighs about three pounds), this twist on the classic burrito bowl features all your favorites—the "rice," the veggies, even the meat.

SERVES 2 TO 3

FOR THE CILANTRO-LIME "RICE"

1 tablespoon extra-virgin olive oil

1 white onion, diced

¼ cup cilantro

Juice of 2 limes

½ teaspoon iodized sea salt

FOR THE FAJITA VEGGIES

1 tablespoon extra-virgin olive oil

1 red onion, slivered

1 red bell pepper, seeded and peeled (optional, Phase 3 only)

1 cup sliced brown mushrooms (like cremini)

2 cups chard, thinly sliced

1 teaspoon cumin

¼ teaspoon iodized sea salt

FOR THE "MEAT"

1 tablespoon extra-virgin olive oil

1 bag Quorn crumbles

½ teaspoon cumin

½ teaspoon paprika

½ teaspoon black pepper

½ teaspoon iodized sea salt

TO ASSEMBLE EACH BOWL

½ cup cilantro lime rice

½ cup fajita veggies

½ cup meat

2 tablespoons Plant Paradox Guacamole (page 259)

1 tablespoon goat's milk cheddar (Trader Joe's or Redwood Hill Farms), shredded (optional)

1 tablespoon goat's milk yogurt (optional)

FOR THE CILANTRO-LIME "RICE"

1. Heat the olive oil over medium heat in a large sauté pan. Add the onion, and cook, stirring occasionally, until onion is tender.

2. Add the cauliflower rice and sauté until tender.

3. Remove from heat, then stir in the cilantro, lime juice, and sea salt. Set aside until ready to serve.

FOR THE FAJITA VEGGIES

1. Heat the olive oil over medium heat in a large sauté pan. Add the onion and cook, stirring occasionally, until onion is tender.

2. Add the pepper and mushrooms, and continue to cook for 3 to 5 minutes.

3. Add the chard, cumin, and sea salt, and cook until chard is wilted.

FOR THE "MEAT"

Heat the olive oil over medium heat in a large skillet. Add the Quorn crumbles and the seasonings and cook, stirring occasionally, until cooked through. If the mixture is browning too fast, reduce heat to low.

TO ASSEMBLE EACH BOWL

Spoon cauliflower rice into the bottom of each bowl. Layer with veggies and meat, then top with top with guacamole. Add cheddar and yogurt if desired. Serve immediately.

Shrimp Poke Bowl

Poke shops are popping up everywhere here in Southern California, and I can see why—the dish, a Hawaiian classic, is incredibly versatile, refreshing, and easy to customize. I make this bowl with cooked wild shrimp, which is widely available, but you can swap in sushi-grade fish if you'd prefer.

SERVES 1

1 tablespoon rice wine vinegar

1 tablespoon coconut aminos

2 tablespoon avocado mayonnaise

1 teaspoon sesame seeds

1 to 2 drops stevia

1 tablespoon diced dried seaweed (nori), crumbled

1 tablespoon sesame oil

1 teaspoon fresh minced ginger

1 clove garlic, minced

3 ounces wild shrimp, deveined, shelled (or leave shells on if you like their lectin-fighting abilities!), and chopped, or hearts of palm

1 cup steamed cauliflower rice

¼ avocado

¼ cup seaweed salad (optional, available at many Japanese markets or in the sushi bar section at your local store)

Sriracha or other hot sauce (optional)

1. Whisk together the rice vinegar, coconut aminos, mayonnaise, sesame seeds, stevia, and seaweed. Set aside.

2. Heat the sesame oil over medium heat in a skillet. Add ginger, garlic, and shrimp. Cook, stirring occasionally, for 2 to 3 minutes, or until shrimp are cooked through.

3. Toss the shrimp together with the sauce.

4. Serve over cauliflower rice, with the avocado and seaweed salad, if using. Drizzle with Sriracha, if desired, and serve.

Egg Roll in a Bowl

I read a lot of food blogs, and one of my favorites is called Peace, Love, and Low Carb, written by Kyndra Holley. This dish is inspired by Kyndra's "Crack Slaw," with a few Plant Paradox–friendly twists.

SERVES 2 TO 4

2 tablespoons sesame oil

3 cloves garlic, minced

1 yellow onion, diced

4 green onions, thinly sliced

1 tablespoon fresh ginger, minced

1 bag Quorn grounds or 1 cup wild-caught shrimp

Iodized sea salt and black pepper, to taste

1 tablespoon garlic chili sauce or Sriracha (use less or more, to taste)

3 cups shredded cabbage

2 cups broccoli slaw (shredded broccoli stalks sold packaged in the produce section)

3 tablespoons coconut aminos

1 tablespoon rice wine vinegar

2 tablespoons toasted sesame seeds

1. Heat the sesame oil in a large sauté pan or wok over medium-high heat.

2. Add the garlic, onion, green onion, and ginger, and cook until the vegetables are soft and fragrant.

3. Add the Quorn grounds or shrimp, salt, pepper, and garlic chili sauce if using, and stir until the Quorn grounds are warmed through or the shrimp has turned light pink.

4. Add the cabbage, broccoli slaw, coconut aminos, rice vinegar, and sesame seeds to the wok, toss until well combined, and cook until cabbage is tender.

5. Serve immediately.

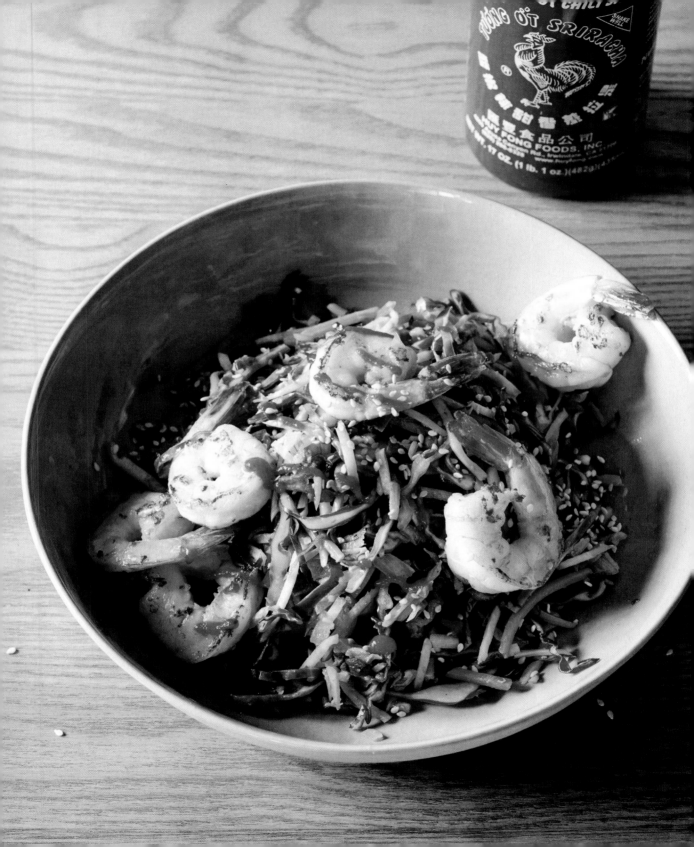

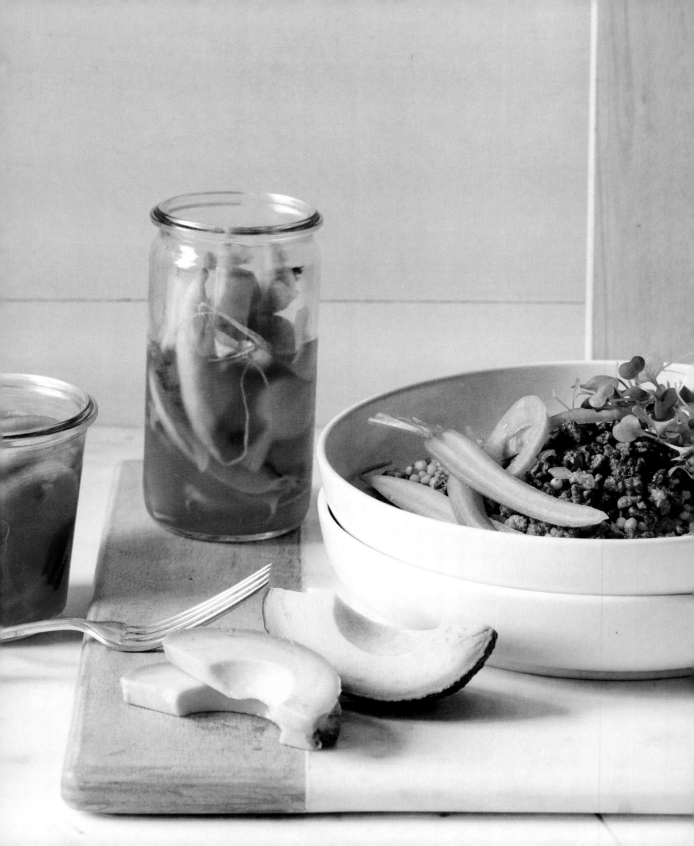

Sorghum Bowl

Sorghum is one of those grains that I *love*, because it's lectin-free and delicious. In fact, I'll sometimes pop sorghum in a pan like popcorn and eat it while watching a movie. But for this recipe, balancing it with creamy avocado and tangy pickled veggies is the way to go.

SERVES 1

1 tablespoon olive oil

½ small yellow onion, minced

1 clove garlic, minced

½ cup Quorn crumbles

1 cup cooked sorghum

¼ cup pickled carrots*

¼ cup pickled beets*

¼ cup pickled onions*

¼ cup pickled radishes*

½ avocado, diced

1. Heat the olive oil in a medium skillet over medium-high heat.

2. Add the onion and sauté 2 to 3 minutes until tender. Add the garlic and sauté an additional minute until fragrant.

3. Add the Quorn crumbles and sorghum and cook, stirring regularly, until flavors meld.

4. Transfer to a serving bowl and top with the pickled veggies and avocado. Serve immediately.

* You can buy pickled vegetables or make your own Quick-Pickled Vegetables (page 208).

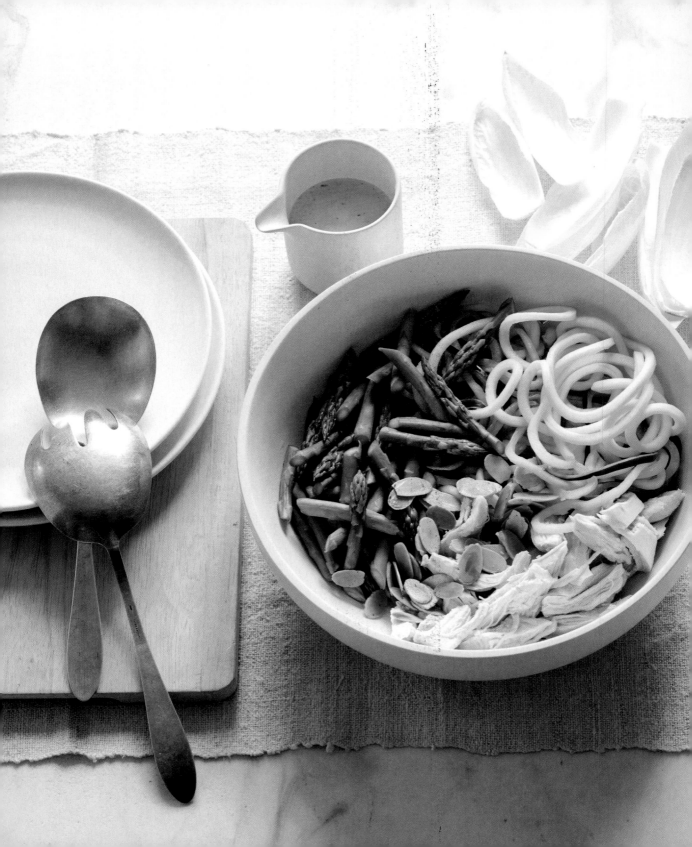

Baby Zucchini Noodles with Creamy Avocado Sauce

This comfort food recipe is made more Plant Paradox–friendly by baby zucchini, which are lighter in lectins than adult zucchini. This dish is perfect for people who love fettucine alfredo—it's got a similar creaminess, as well as plenty of gut-healthy vegetables to add crunch. Thanks to Irina Skoeries of Catalyst Cuisine for the recipe!

SERVES 2 TO 3

1 tablespoon avocado oil

4 ounces boneless, skinless chicken breast (pastured), cut into strips (optional)

¼ teaspoon iodized sea salt

¼ teaspoon freshly cracked black pepper

1 large endive, shredded

12 fresh asparagus spears, cut into 2- to 3-inch pieces

8 baby zucchinis, spiralized,* set aside

¼ cup blanched almonds, chopped (slivered almonds work as well)

FOR THE AVOCADO SAUCE

1 large ripe avocado

½ cup full-fat coconut milk

½ cup water

Juice of 1 lemon

½ teaspoon salt

¼ teaspoon freshly cracked black pepper

1 teaspoon fresh thyme

1. Heat the avocado oil on medium-high heat and add the chicken (or move to step 2, if not using chicken). Sprinkle with salt and pepper and sauté until cooked through, about 5 to 6 minutes.

2. Add the endive and asparagus and continue cooking until the veggies become tender, about 3 to 4 minutes.

3. While the chicken and vegetables are cooking, add all the ingredients for the avocado sauce to a food processor fitted with an S-blade and process until smooth and creamy.

4. Add the reserved zucchini to the chicken (if using) and vegetables, and mix well. The heat from this alone will be enough to cook the zucchini and make it nice and soft.

5. Stir in avocado sauce, followed by chopped almonds, and serve.

You can cut zucchini into thin strips with a mandoline or a sharp knife if you don't have a spiralizer.

Creamy Shrimp and Kale Spaghetti

Sometimes you just want pasta for dinner—we all do. And what's better than a creamy spaghetti dish that you don't feel guilty about eating? You can make this dish without the shrimp if you'd prefer to keep it vegetarian—it is a filling meal even without the additional protein.

SERVES 2

¼ cup extra-virgin olive oil

1 brown onion, thinly sliced

3 cloves garlic, thinly sliced

6 ounces wild-caught shrimp, deveined (optional)

2 cups thinly sliced kale

1 cup unsweetened coconut cream

Juice of 1 lemon

¼ cup grated Parmigiano-Reggiano or 2 tablespoons nutritional yeast

FOR THE MIRACLE NOODLES, COOKED THE GUNDRY WAY

1 package Miracle Noodles spaghetti

Iodized sea salt, to taste.

1. Heat the olive oil in a large skillet over medium heat.

2. Add the onion, and cook for 3 to 4 minutes, until tender and translucent.

3. Add garlic and shrimp (if using), and cook an additional 2 minutes, until shrimp are pink and garlic is fragrant.

4. Reduce heat to low and add the kale, coconut cream, and lemon. Cook until the kale is wilted, then whisk in the Parmigiano or yeast.

5. Cook for 3 to 4 minutes, then add prepared Miracle Noodles. Cook an additional 2 minutes, then serve.

FOR THE MIRACLE NOODLES, COOKED THE GUNDRY WAY

1. Bring a pot of salted water to a boil.

2. Remove your noodles from the package and rinse under cold running water for 2 to 3 minutes.

3. Transfer noodles to boiling water and cook 2 to 3 minutes.

4. Transfer to a dry pan and cook over medium-low heat, stirring to dry out the noodles.

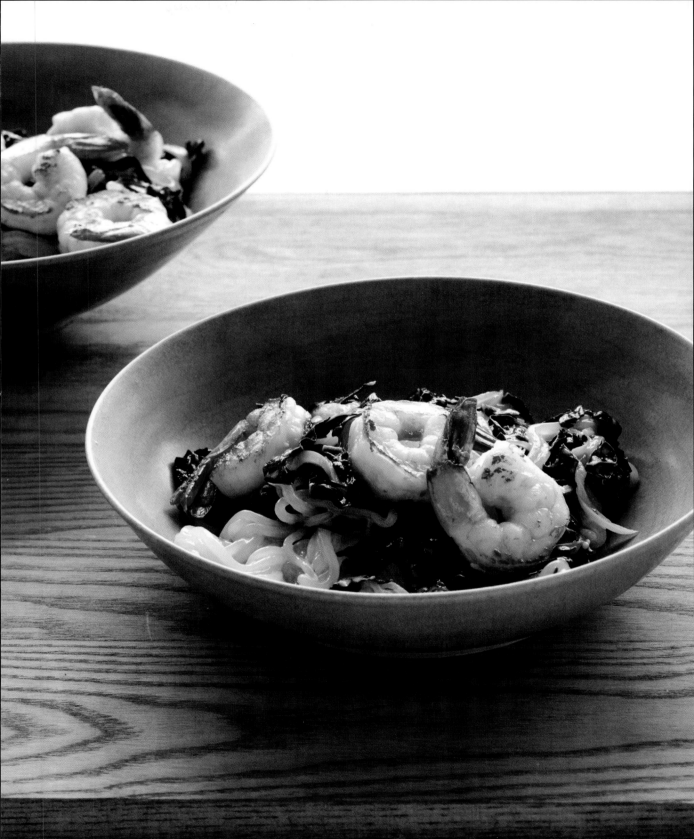

Not Bad Pad Thai

I offered a pad Thai recipe on my YouTube channel that was so popular, I knew I wanted to include a version of it in this book. I think this dish is even better than the original! It comes together quickly for a filling, flavorful dinner.

SERVES 2

2 tablespoons olive oil

1 tablespoon sesame oil

2 garlic cloves

6 ounces wild shrimp, shells off (optional)

½ cup broccoli slaw (optional)

1 omega-3 or pastured egg or VeganEgg

½ cup basil leaves, chopped

One 8-ounce package fettuccine-style Miracle Noodles*

Juice of 2 limes

4 tablespoons chopped dry roasted macadamia nuts

1 to 2 tablespoons fish sauce or coconut aminos

1 tablespoon unsweetened, unseasoned rice vinegar

Pinch of stevia

1 teaspoon paprika

1. Heat the oils in a large skillet over high heat, but not hot enough to cause them to smoke.

2. Add the garlic, and stir briefly, then add the shrimp and broccoli slaw (if using), and stir for an additional minute.

3. Add egg, and stir for another minute, until cooked.

4. Add the basil, noodles, lime juice, macadamia nuts, fish sauce or coconut aminos, rice vinegar, stevia, and paprika, and stir-fry for about 3 more minutes, until the shrimp is opaque. Remove from heat and serve immediately.

See page 156 for preparation instructions.

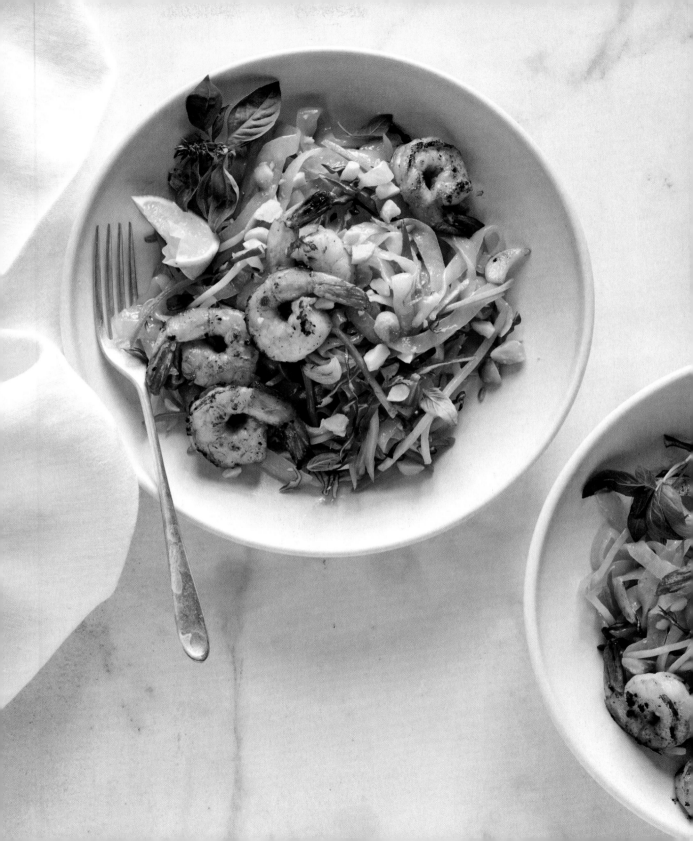

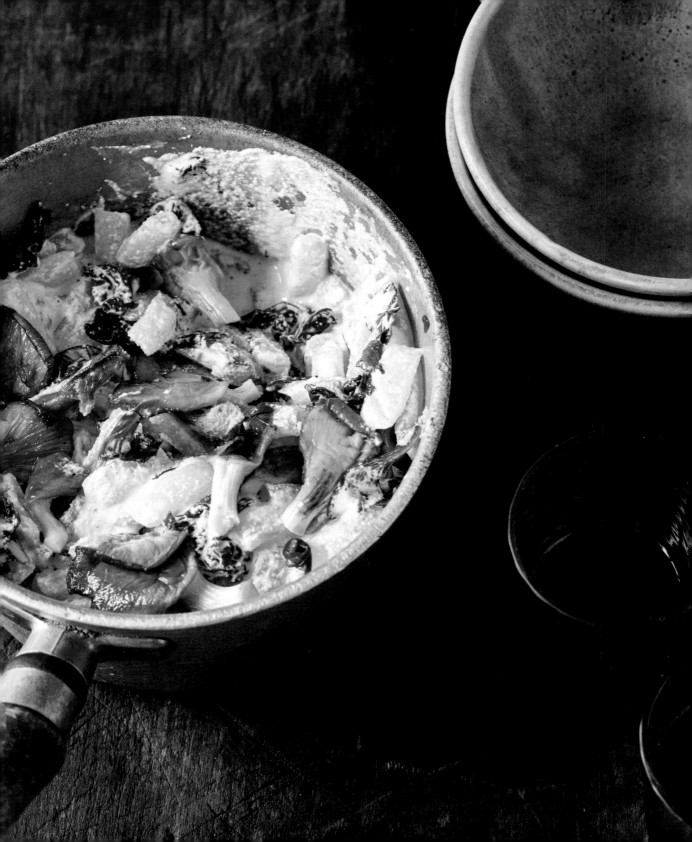

Truffled Mushroom Mac and Cheese

This recipe came from our second-place winner in the Plant Paradox recipe contest, Jenni Schultz. It's a delicious, completely vegan mac and cheese that's just as good as the dairy-laden version, but way better for your gut! Jenni's tried-and-true recipe uses Miracle Noodles, but I've also used this sauce with sweet potato noodles and Capello Almond noodles, and it's equally delicious.

SERVES 1

FOR THE CHEESE SAUCE*

1 cup raw macadamia nuts, soaked for 8 hours or overnight

¾ cup water

Juice from ½ lemon

¼ cup nutritional yeast

1 teaspoon iodized sea salt

½ teaspoon smoked paprika

⅛ teaspoon powdered mustard

½ clove garlic

Pinch of black pepper

FOR THE MAC AND CHEESE

1 package ziti-style Miracle Noodles or fettucine, cut into small pieces

2 teaspoons buffalo ghee or avocado oil

2 large oyster mushrooms, roughly chopped

¼ cup cheese sauce

1 handful fresh spinach

Iodized sea salt and black pepper to taste

Nutritional yeast to sprinkle

½ teaspoon truffle oil

1. First, make the cheese sauce: Place all ingredients in a high-speed blender such as a Vitamix or a Blendtec or in the work bowl of a food processor fitted with an S-blade.

2. Blend on high until smooth. You may need to add more water, 1 tablespoon at a time, if the mixture is too thick.

3. Prepare the Miracle Noodle ziti the Gundry way (page 156). Set aside.

4. In a small-to-medium saucepan over medium heat, heat the buffalo ghee or avocado oil, and sauté the oyster mushrooms.

5. Once soft, add the noodles, cheese sauce, and spinach, and heat on medium-to-low heat until the spinach has wilted.

6. Add the salt, pepper, nutritional yeast, and truffle oil, and stir to combine.

* The cheese sauce will make enough for a little more than 4 servings of the mac and cheese. You can store in a glass container in the fridge for 5 days, or in the freezer for up to 2 months. If freezing, let thaw slowly in the refrigerator to maintain consistency.

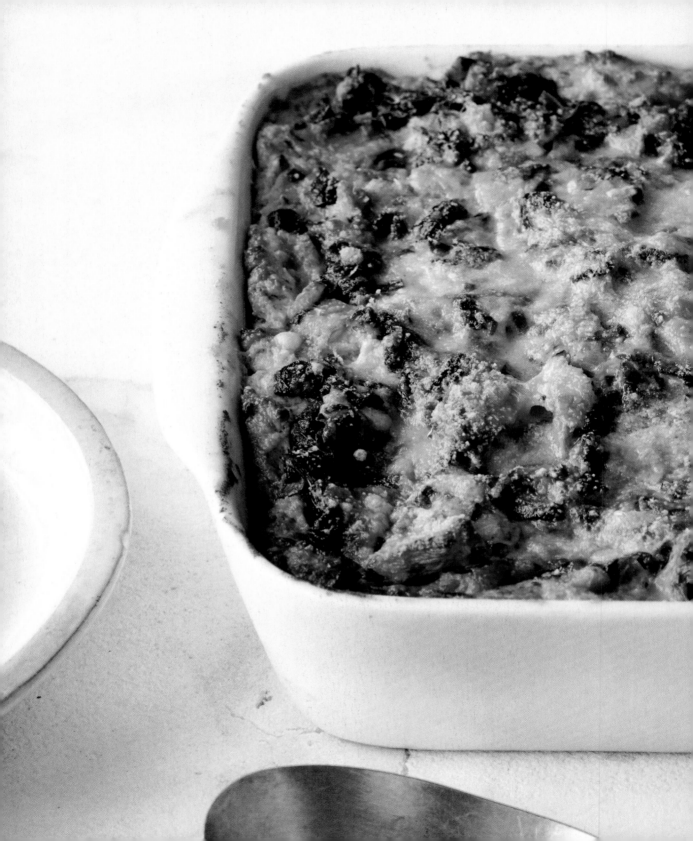

chapter nine

Main Dishes

Superfood Salad

Sometimes you need a healthy helping of something green, and this salad fits the bill. It's tasty and filling, and it keeps well in the fridge. To take it to go, I suggest adding the dressing and the heartier ingredients to the bottom of a large Mason jar, and piling the greens on top. To serve, just invert it onto a plate and—voilà—instant dressed salad!

SERVES 1

2 cups baby kale and arugula

¼ cup artichoke hearts, frozen and thawed, minced (canned will work in a pinch, just make sure they have no sugar added, and rinse them well before using)

½ cup broccoli slaw

¼ cup raw red beets, shredded

¼ cup radishes, sliced

2 tablespoons Classic Balsamic Vinaigrette (page 260)

¼ cup pomegranate seeds (if in season, September through January)

½ avocado, diced

1 omega-3 or pastured egg, hard-boiled and crumbled (optional)

1. In a large salad bowl, place the greens, artichoke hearts, broccoli slaw, beets, radishes, and vinaigrette. Toss, using salad tongs or clean hands, until well dressed.

2. Transfer to plate, and garnish with the pomegranate seeds, avocado, and egg, if using.

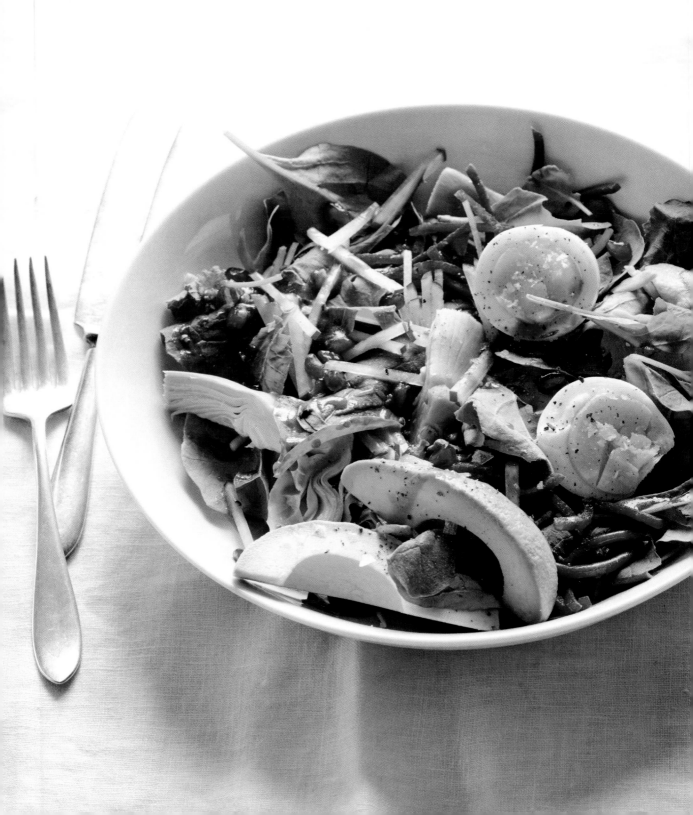

Jonathan Waxman's Kale Salad

This salad recipe came to us from chef Jonathan Waxman of Barbuto in New York City, and it's just about the best kale salad on the planet. If you're worried about the anchovies, don't be! They make the dressing salty, not fishy.

SERVES 4

1 pound fresh kale, baby if possible, or the youngest dinosaur kale available

4 leaves basil

2 cloves garlic, smashed

2 salt-cured anchovies, rinsed and filleted*

1 egg yolk

1 tablespoon Dijon mustard

1 tablespoon lemon juice (about ¼ of a large lemon)

¼ cup extra-virgin olive oil

Iodized sea salt and pepper, to taste

1 ounce grated Pecorino-Romano cheese*

1 tablespoon finely chopped toasted hazelnuts

1. Wash the kale well and dry in a salad spinner. On a wood cutting board, cut the kale into ribbons as thin as possible. Place the kale in a salad bowl.

2. On the cutting board, finely mince the basil, garlic, and anchovies.

3. In another bowl, add the basil and garlic mixture, egg, mustard, and lemon juice. Use a whisk and mix well. Drizzle in the olive oil and whisk briskly to combine.

4. Pour dressing over the kale, enough to coat the leaves well.

5. Using as much force as possible, crush the kale and dressing with a wooden spoon. (At Barbuto they use their hands, but with gloves of course!) Add a pinch of sea salt and black pepper.

6. Sprinkle with the cheese and nuts.

7. Toss well, taste for seasoning, and serve.

To make this salad vegan: Omit the anchovies, egg, and cheese, and whisk 2 tablespoons of nutritional yeast into the dressing.

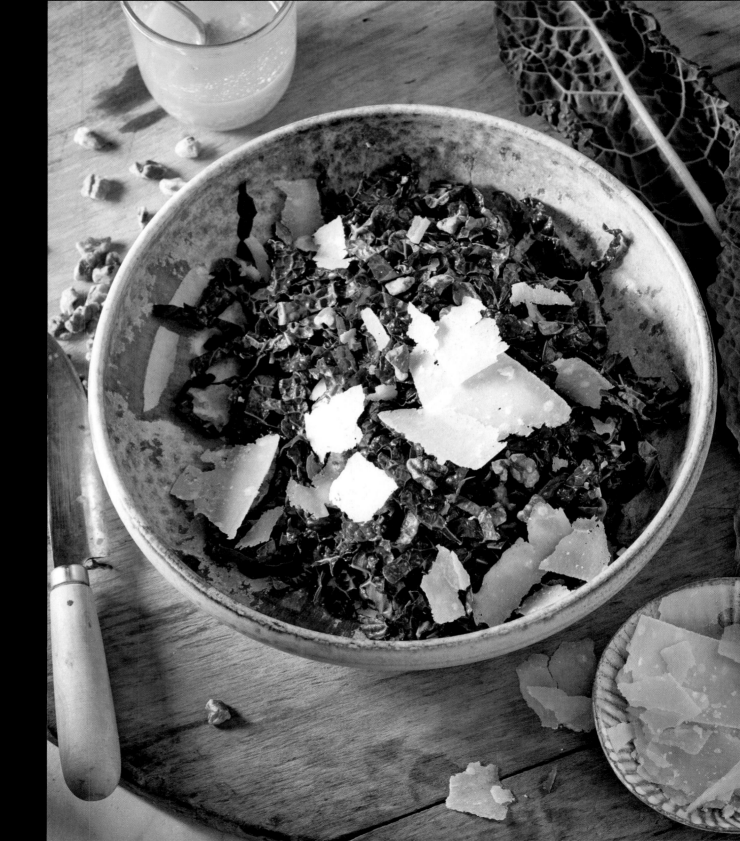

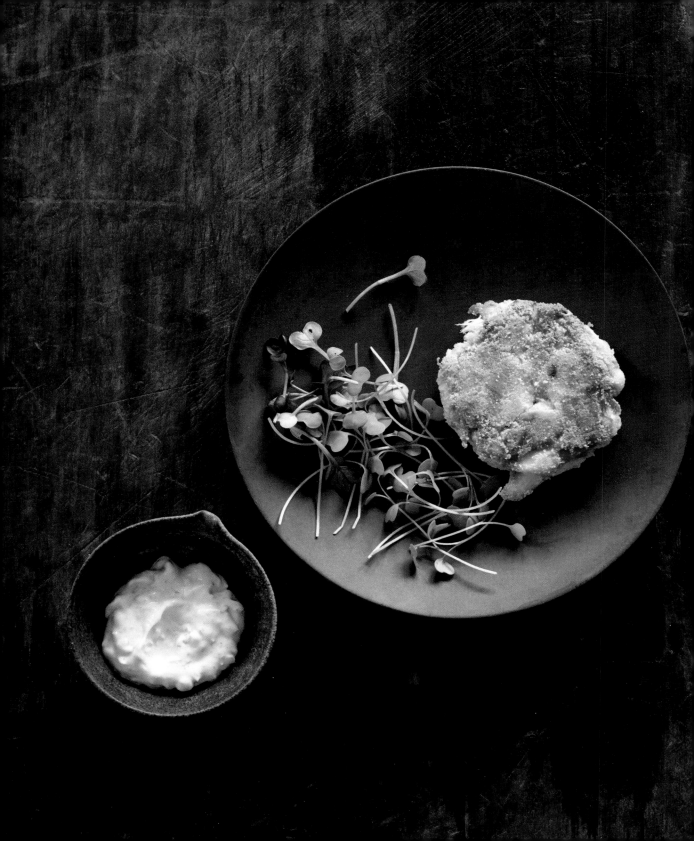

Crab Cakes

I love a good crab cake, but I'll confess: I often make the vegetarian version of these even when I have access to high-quality lump crabmeat. It's easy, affordable, delicious, and so close in flavor to the real thing that I've fooled my own dinner guests!

SERVES 2

FOR DIPPING SAUCE

½ cup avocado mayonnaise, such as Primal Kitchen

1 tablespoon capers

1 teaspoon diced onion

1 tablespoon diced green olives

Zest of 1 lemon

FOR CRAB CAKES

14 ounces of lump crab meat *or* 14 ounces of hearts of palm (frozen, jarred, or canned and packed in brine, not sugar) drained and finely chopped

2 celery stalks, diced

½ yellow onion, diced

2 cloves garlic, crushed

1 teaspoon Old Bay seasoning

2 tablespoons cassava flour

1 omega-3 or pastured egg or VeganEgg

¼ cup blanched almond flour (Bob's Red Mill makes a great one, available at most grocery stores)

3 tablespoons avocado oil

1. First, make the sauce: combine all the ingredients in a small bowl. Cover and refrigerate until needed.

2. In a large bowl, combine the crab (or hearts of palm), celery, onion, garlic, Old Bay, cassava flour, and egg. The mixture should easily form cakes between your hands. If it's falling apart, add more cassava, 1 teaspoon at a time, until it comes together.

3. Form the crab mixture into four evenly sized cakes. Gently pat almond flour onto the outside of each one, then refrigerate for 15 to 20 minutes, until cakes hold together.

4. Heat avocado oil over medium-high heat in a large skillet. Cook crab cakes until browned, about 3 to 4 minutes. Gently flip and cook for an additional 3 to 4 minutes.

5. Reduce heat to low, and continue to cook until a sharp knife inserted into the center of one cake comes out hot (1 to 2 minutes more).

6. Serve with sauce.

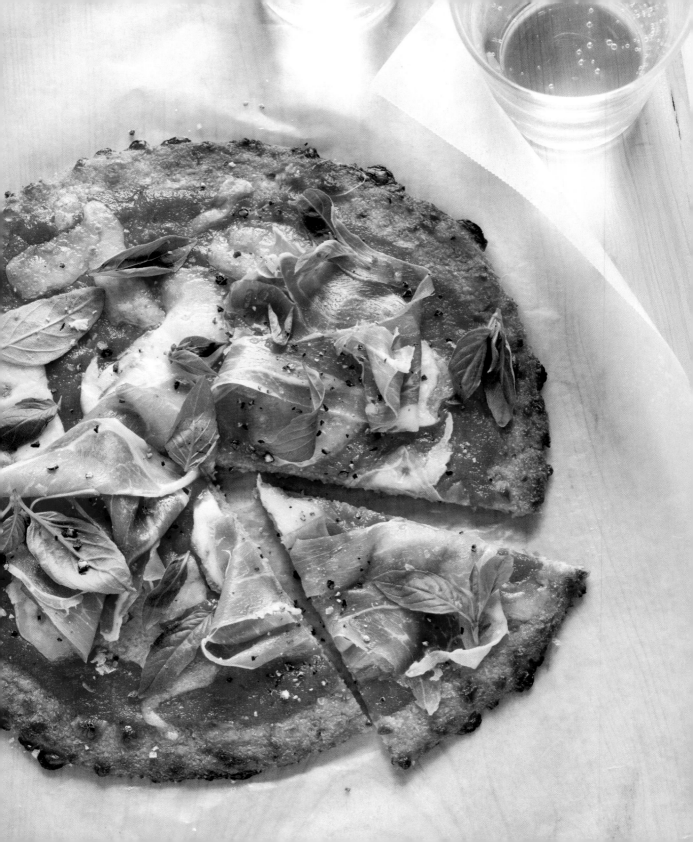

Pizza with Cauliflower Crust

Pizza on the Plant Paradox plan?! It's true, you're not seeing things. This recipe comes from our friend Tara Lazar, a local chef here in Palm Springs. I think her cauliflower crust is the best I've ever had. If you're on Phase 3, try making a tomato sauce with peeled, seeded tomatoes to enjoy the full pizza experience!

MAKES TWO 8-INCH CRUSTS

butter or coconut oil, for greasing baking sheet

2¾ cups cauliflower flour (page 172)

¼ cup almond flour

2 tablespoons tapioca flour

1 cup shredded buffalo mozzarella cheese

1½ omega-3 or pastured eggs or VeganEggs*

TOPPING IDEAS

Classic Basil Pesto (page 258), prosciutto, and buffalo mozzarella

Classic Basil Pesto and caramelized onions

Sheep's milk ricotta, lemon zest, sliced figs

Addicitve Caramelized Onion Bourbon Jam (page 254), figs, and balsamic glaze

Phase 3 Tomato Sauce (page 173), buffalo mozzarella, basil

1. Preheat the oven to 300°F. Grease a sheet of parchment paper with butter or coconut oil.

2. Place all the ingredients in a large bowl. Using your hands, mix well to combine.

3. Divide the crust in half, forming two balls.

4. Place each ball onto the sheet of buttered (or coconut-oiled) parchment paper, and flatten with greased hands into an 8-inch round, making sure the crusts are even with no holes.

5. Bake for 15 minutes, turning the crusts halfway through to be sure they are cooked evenly.

6. Remove crusts, and increase oven heat to 350°F.

7. Top with desired toppings, then return to oven and bake until edges begin to crisp.

For half an egg, scramble a whole egg, and use half by weight.

(continued)

Cauliflower Flour

3 medium-size cauliflower
stalks, leaves removed

¾ cups grated Parmigiano-
Reggiano

1½ teaspoon garlic powder

1½ teaspoon onion powder

Salt and pepper, to taste

Juicer Method: Cut the cauliflower into medium-size chunks and pass through a juicer so that most of the liquid is removed from the pulp.

Discard juice and save pulp. Move on to step 1, below.

Food Processor Method: Cut the cauliflower, place in a food processor, and pulse until broken into tiny pieces (smaller than grains of rice).

Transfer the cauliflower to a clean kitchen towel, and squeeze pulp, trying to extract as much water as possible.

Transfer the pulp into a microwave-safe bowl. Microwave in 15- to 20-second increments (your goal here is to start to dry out the cauliflower).

Strain, and squeeze through cloth again to extract more water before moving on to step 1, below.

1. Preheat the oven to 350°F.

2. Spread the pulp on a parchment-lined sheet tray and transfer to the oven. Cook for 10 to 15 minutes, keeping a close eye on the cauliflower. You want the volume of the cauliflower pulp to reduce by half, but you do *not* want the cauliflower to burn. If it is browning too quickly, reduce heat to 300°F.

3. Once reduced, add the Parmigiano, garlic, onion powder, salt, and pepper.

4. Remove from the oven and let cool to room temperature.

Phase 3 Tomato Sauce

¼ cup extra-virgin olive oil

1 large onion, diced

3 cloves garlic, minced

8 large ripe tomatoes, peeled with a serrated peeler, seeds removed, or use boxed tomatoes, like Pomi

1 tablespoon red wine vinegar

Salt and pepper to taste

1. Heat the oil in a large sauce pot over medium-high heat. Add the onions and cook, stirring regularly, until translucent. Add the garlic and cook an additional minute or 2.

2. Add the tomatoes, vinegar, and a bit of salt and pepper, and reduce heat to low.

3. Cook, covered, for 15 to 20 minutes, until tomatoes begin to break down.

4. Transfer the sauce to a blender (or use an immersion blender) to blend, then continue to cook, uncovered, for 15 to 20 minutes.

5. Cook until thickened, stirring occasionally.

Halibut with Mushroom Ragout and Lentils

This recipe is courtesy of my friend a James Beard Award–winning chef Jimmy Schmidt. It may seem a little complicated at first, but it's one of those recipes that's easier than it looks. I suggest doubling or tripling the lentils and storing leftovers in the fridge or freezer—it makes a great weeknight side dish or even a full meal.

SERVES 4

FOR THE LENTILS

2 tablespoons avocado oil

½ cup shallots, peeled and finely diced

2 cloves of garlic, peeled and sliced paper-thin

1 cup lentils

2½ cups mushroom stock or Vegetable Stock (page 265)

2 tablespoons dried porcini mushroom powder, finely ground (make your own by pulsing dried porcinis in a spice grinder)*

2 tablespoons agave syrup

Iodized sea salt, to taste

Freshly ground black pepper, to taste

FOR THE RAGOUT

2 tablespoons avocado oil

½ pound chanterelle mushrooms, stems trimmed and caps torn into large pieces; cut 2 tablespoons of the firmest mushrooms into fine strips and reserve for the salad**

Small bunch of scallions, green tops cut on angle for garnish, white bottoms sliced thin for sauté

1. Preheat the oven to 425°F.

2. Prepare the lentils: In a large skillet over medium heat, add the avocado oil and the shallots. Cook, stirring occasionally, until translucent.

3. Add the garlic, lentils, stock, porcini powder, and agave syrup, bringing to a short boil. Season generously with sea salt and pepper. Transfer this mixture to your pressure cooker, and lock down the lid. Pressure-cook at high for 15 minutes. Remove from heat and allow the pressure cooker to release pressure naturally, about 10 minutes.

4. Make the ragout: Add 2 tablespoons of the avocado oil to a large skillet over high heat. Cook the large pieces of the chanterelles and the scallion whites until browned—about 5 minutes. Add the white wine and a drizzle of balsamic vinegar, cooking until reduced, about 2 minutes. Add the cooked lentils and the scallion greens, stirring to combine. Adjust the seasoning with sea salt and pepper. Stir in the Parmigiano cheese.

5. Prepare the fish: Season the halibut surfaces with coriander, sea salt, and pepper. In a medium skillet, heat a few drops of the avocado oil over high heat. Add the halibut to sear, about 2 minutes, then turn the filets over.

(continued)

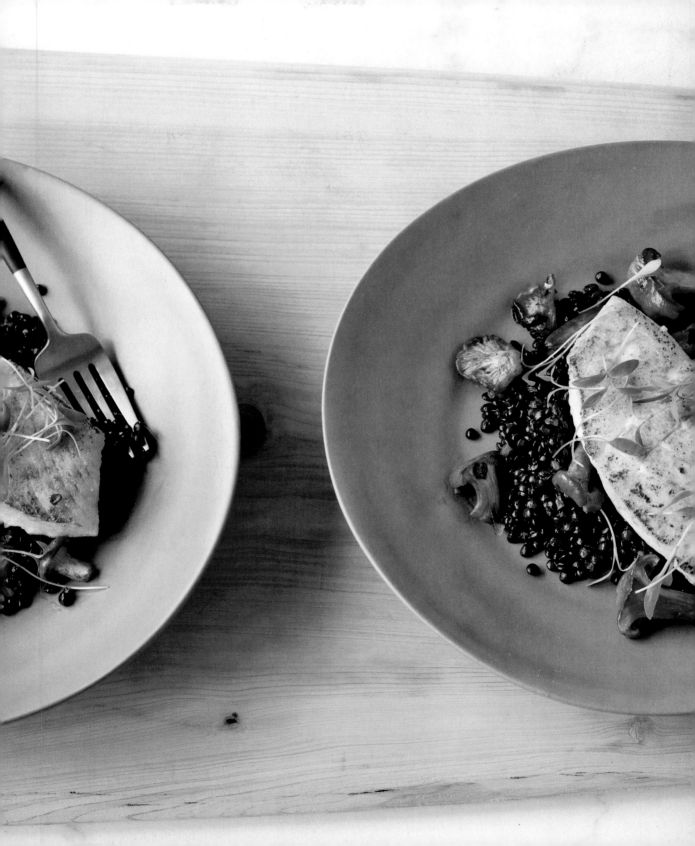

½ cup dry white wine

Drizzle of balsamic vinegar

2 tablespoons Parmigiano-Reggiano, finely grated

FOR THE FISH

2 tablespoons of ground coriander seed

Iodized sea salt, to taste

Freshly ground black pepper, to taste

4 halibut center filets (thicker), 4 to 5 ounces each

½ cup cilantro

Transfer to the lower rack of your oven to finish cooking, about 6 minutes, depending on the thickness of the filets and your desired degree of doneness.

6. To serve: Spoon the lentil ragout with mushrooms to the center of your plate and position the halibut on top. In a small bowl, combine the cilantro and raw julienne of chanterelles, tossing with a little sea salt and pepper. Place atop the halibut. Serve and enjoy.

If you can't find porcinis or porcini powder, pick the most fragrant dried mushrooms you can find, and grind them.

**If I'm often able to find chanterelles in Whole Foods or at a local farmer's markets. If unavailable, try porcinis, trumpets, or shiitakes.*

Thai Lemongrass "Meat" Balls

Meatballs without the meat? Sure, it's absolutely possible—this recipe uses Quorn grounds in place of meat, although you could also use ground, grass-fed, pastured beef if you prefer. If using Quorn, make sure not to grind the grounds too small, or you'll lose the texture and get a gummy meatball. Want to keep it vegan? Skip the Quorn grounds and triple the sweet potatoes.

SERVES 4

1 tablespoon sesame oil

1 tablespoon fresh ginger, minced

1 clove garlic, minced

1 stalk lemongrass, dry layers removed, thinly sliced

1 teaspoon Thai red curry paste

1 bag Quorn grounds, thawed, or 12 ounces grass-fed ground beef

1 small sweet potato, baked, skin removed, and mashed (about ½ cup)

1 omega-3 or pastured egg or VeganEgg

2 tablespoon cassava flour

2 tablespoons avocado oil

1 can coconut milk

1 tablespoon coconut aminos

Steamed cauliflower rice, for serving

1. Heat a small skillet over medium-high heat. Add the sesame oil, ginger, garlic, and lemongrass, and sauté, stirring frequently, until very fragrant, about 2 minutes.

2. Add the curry paste, and cook an additional minute.

3. Transfer the mixture to the work bowl of a food processor, add the Quorn and sweet potato, and pulse until well combined (mixture should be a little chunky).

4. Transfer to a bowl, and add the egg and cassava flour. Mixture should be able to be formed into balls. If too loose, add more flour, one teaspoon at a time, until it becomes more cohesive.

5. Scoop the mixture into tablespoon-size balls, using your hands or an ice cream scoop. Refrigerate for 20 minutes.

6. Heat the avocado oil in a large skillet over medium-high heat. Once the balls are chilled, transfer them to the pan and cook, stirring occasionally, until browned on all sides, 5 to 7 minutes.

7. Add the coconut milk and coconut aminos, and continue to cook, 5 minutes, until sauce has thickened slightly.

8. Serve over steamed cauliflower rice.

Moroccan-Spiced Chicken with Millet Tabbouleh

I'm mixing metaphors a bit with this dish—a little Moroccan inspired, a little Middle-Eastern inspired. But the thing is, the flavors taste delicious together. This twist on classic tabbouleh is wonderful paired with grilled seafood, meat, or tempeh, and it's great on its own too!

SERVES 4

FOR THE CHICKEN

2 cups coconut yogurt, plain

Juice of 1 lemon

Zest of 1 lemon

Zest of 1 orange

½ teaspoon cinnamon

½ teaspoon cumin

½ teaspoon paprika

½ teaspoon black pepper

½ teaspoon turmeric

½ teaspoon iodized sea salt

4 pasture-raised chicken thighs*

FOR THE TABBOULEH

2 cups cooked millet

½ cup minced parsley

½ cup minced mint

¼ cup minced dill

1 teaspoon iodized sea salt

1 tablespoon extra-virgin olive oil

Juice of 1 lemon

¼ cup red wine vinegar

1. Marinate the chicken: In a large ziplock bag, combine the yogurt, lemon juice, lemon zest, orange zest, and spices. Add the chicken, and marinate for at least 1 hour. (If using tempeh, use the same marinade, but for 30 minutes.)

2. Preheat the oven to 375°F. Prepare a broiler pan or a sheet tray with wire rack by spraying with oil. Set aside.

3. Make the tabbouleh: Combine all ingredients in a large bowl, and stir well. Let the flavors meld for at least 20 minutes (which is perfect, since you need that time to cook the chicken).

4. Remove chicken (or tempeh) from marinade, pat dry with paper towels, and arrange on the prepared baking sheet. If your chicken has skin, place it skin-side down.

5. Bake the chicken for 20 to 25 minutes, then flip and bake for an additional 10 to 15 minutes, skin side up, until meat has reached 160°F and skin is crisp. Remove from heat, and let rest 5 minutes before serving.

If using tempeh: Bake for 12 to 15 minutes, flipping occasionally, until crispy. Remove from heat and serve immediately.

To make it vegetarian, use about a pound of tempeh, cut into thick slices.

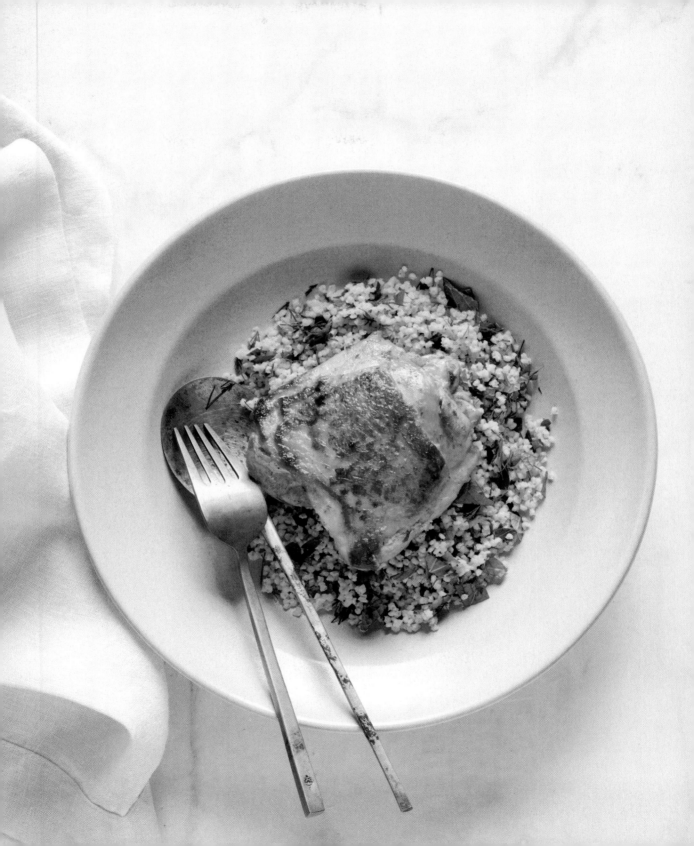

Cauliflower Rice Risotto

One of my favorite things about cauliflower rice is the way it absorbs flavor from the foods you combine with it. This recipe is no exception—the cauliflower takes on the flavor of the mushrooms and coconut cream, resulting in a dish that's rich and flavorful.

SERVES 8

¼ cup avocado oil

6 cups assorted mushrooms

2 medium leeks, rinsed and finely sliced

¼ cup minced shallots

1 16-ounce package cauliflower rice

3 tablespoons arrowroot starch

16 ounces mushroom broth or Bone Broth (page 257)

1 can coconut cream

Juice of 1 lemon

Zest of 1 lemon

¼ cup nutritional yeast or grated Parmigiano-Reggiano cheese

Salt and pepper, to taste

1. Heat a dry pan on high. Add oil to hot pan.

2. Sauté the mushrooms until golden brown (10 minutes, stirring infrequently—let them brown!)

3. Add the leeks, shallots, and a small pinch of salt, and cook until translucent, 4 to 5 minutes.

4. Add the cauliflower rice and sauté for about 5 minutes, then add the arrowroot and stir for about 1 minute.

5. Add the mushroom broth or bone broth, and bring the risotto to a boil—it should start to thicken fairly quickly (2 to 3 minutes).

6. Once boiling and thickened, add the coconut cream, and reduce heat so the mixture is barely simmering.

7. Add the lemon juice, lemon zest, and nutritional yeast or grated Parmigiano-Reggiano, and season to taste. Serve warm.

Spinach Artichoke Lasagna

I love lasagna, but the ingredients read like a list of forbidden foods: pasta, tomato sauce, ricotta cheese. Luckily, you don't need any of those to make a delicious lasagna. I've found that thinly-sliced sweet potatoes work as a perfect substitute for noodles. Beyond that, the flavor possibilities are endless!

SERVES 8

Olive oil spray, plus more for baking dish

¼ cup extra-virgin olive oil

2 cups artichoke hearts (frozen and thawed is best, canned or jarred are okay too, provided they are packed in brine), finely chopped

4 cups baby spinach, rinsed

1 cup cremini mushrooms, finely chopped

1 teaspoon iodized sea salt

½ teaspoon black pepper

½ teaspoon fresh thyme

Zest of 1 lemon

1 tablespoon fresh rosemary, minced

1 can unsweetened coconut cream

2 cups sheep's or goat's milk ricotta, or 3 cups coconut yogurt

2 omega-3 or pastured eggs or VeganEggs

1 cup Classic Basil Pesto (page 258)

1 teaspoon garlic powder

1 teaspoon paprika

¼ cup Parmesan cheese (optional), plus additional to sprinkle on top

1 large sweet potato, thinly sliced (as lasagna noodles; using a mandoline helps)

1. Preheat the oven to 375°F. Spray a 9 × 13-inch baking dish with olive oil and set aside.

2. In a large sauté pan, heat the olive oil over medium-high heat.

3. Add the artichokes, spinach, and mushrooms, and cook, stirring frequently, until tender.

4. Add the salt, pepper, thyme, lemon zest, and rosemary, and cook an additional 3 minutes.

5. Add the coconut cream, reduce heat to low, and let simmer for 10 minutes, while you make the cheese mixture.

6. In a large bowl, combine the ricotta or yogurt, eggs, pesto, garlic powder, paprika, and cheese. Set aside.

7. Spoon half a cup of artichoke mixture into the baking dish, followed by the first layer of sweet potato "noodles."

8. Top with 1 cup of the ricotta mixture and another half cup of the artichoke mixture. Continue to layer until pan is full.

9. Sprinkle the top of the lasagna with the Parmigiano-Reggiano, and cover pan with foil.

10. Bake for 35 to 40 minutes, then remove the foil and bake an additional 15 minutes, until cheese is golden brown.

11. Remove from heat and let rest 10 minutes before serving.

Root Vegetable Lasagna

Pasta sauce without tomatoes? Sure, if it's a rich, highly seasoned root vegetable sauce. When I make this dish for myself, I use about 5 times the garlic, but I'm an addict. If you're hooked on garlic like me, try using a whole head instead of just a couple of cloves.

SERVES 8

¼ cup olive oil, plus more for baking dish

1 yellow onion, diced

1 cup diced parsnips

1 cup diced celery root

1 cup diced rutabaga or turnips

1 sprig rosemary, leaves minced

2 garlic cloves, peeled and minced

1 teaspoon iodized sea salt

½ teaspoon black pepper

½ cup water

½ cup coconut milk

2 cups goat's or sheep's milk ricotta or 3 cups coconut yogurt

½ teaspoon dried oregano

1 lemon, zested and juiced

1 cup loosely packed basil, julienned

2 omega-3 or pastured eggs or VeganEggs

1 large sweet potato, thinly sliced (as lasagna noodles; using a mandoline helps)

½ cup grated Parmigiano-Reggiano

1. Preheat the oven to 375°F. Spray a 9 × 13-inch baking dish with oil, and set aside.

2. First, make your sauce: Heat olive oil in a large saucepan over medium-high heat.

3. Add the onion, and cook 2 to 3 minutes, until translucent.

4. Add the parsnips, celery root, and rutabaga or turnips, as well as rosemary and garlic, and cook for 15 to 20 minutes, stirring frequently, until vegetables are tender.

5. Add the salt and pepper and blend using an immersion blender (or transfer to a blender), and process until smooth. Sauce should be consistency of thick tomato sauce. If too thick, add water, a little at a time. Whisk in coconut milk and set aside.

6. In a large bowl, combine the ricotta or coconut yogurt, oregano, lemon zest and juice, basil, and the eggs. Set aside.

7. Spoon half a cup of the root veggie sauce into the base of your baking dish, and layer on one layer of the thin-sliced sweet potato "noodles."

8. Top with half a cup of the ricotta mixture, then repeat until pan is full. (It will take three or four layers.)

9. Sprinkle the top of the lasagna with the Parmigiano-Reggiano, and cover the pan with foil.

10. Bake for 35 to 40 minutes, then remove foil and bake for an additional 15 minutes, until cheese is golden brown.

11. Remove from heat and let rest 10 minutes before serving.

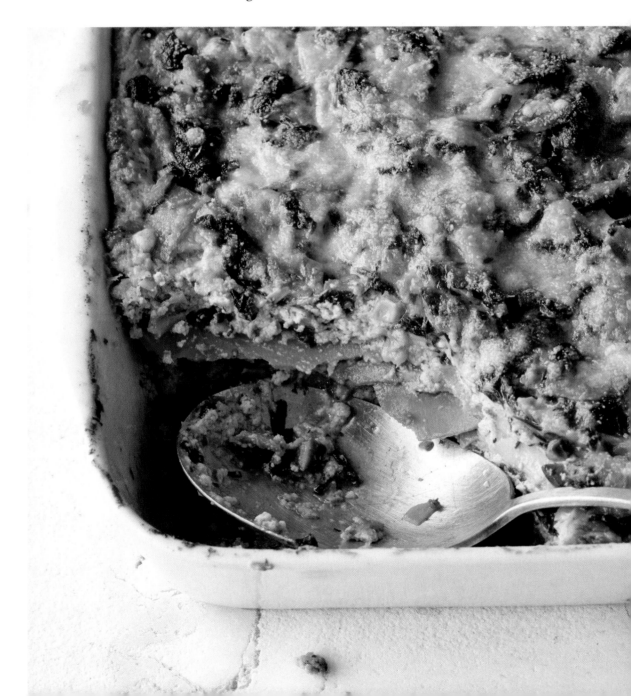

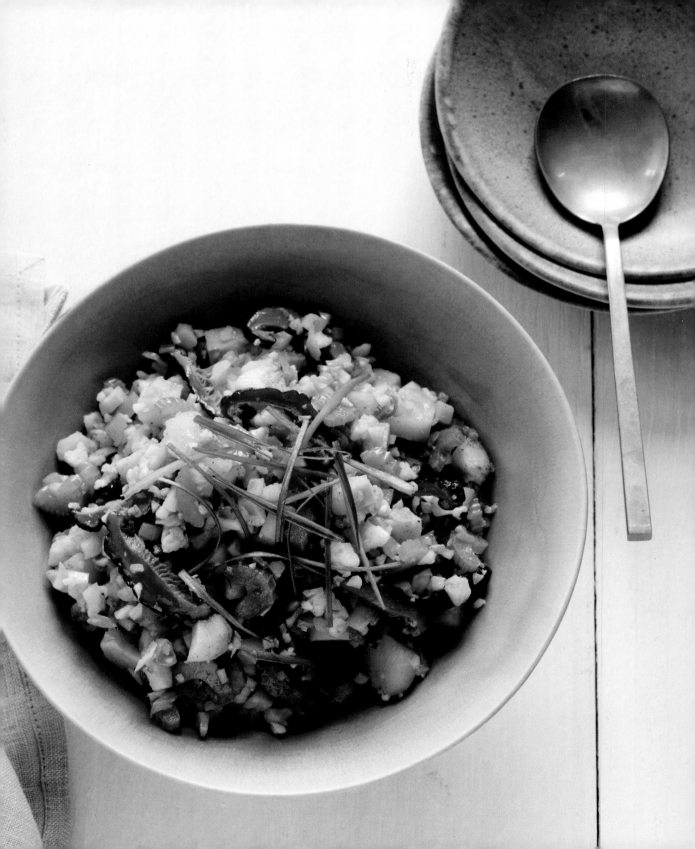

Cauliflower-Ginger Fried Rice

I used to love ordering fried rice when I'd get takeout, and I missed it once I went lectin-free. This fragrant dish, scented with ginger, garlic, and onion, offers the same flavors as your favorite takeout, but is a lot better for you, and keeps your gut happy. It also reheats well, so consider making a double batch if you want leftovers.

SERVES 6 TO 8

2½ tablespoons sesame oil

1 medium yellow onion, diced

1 1-inch piece ginger root, peeled and minced

2 cloves garlic, minced

8 to 12 dried shiitake mushrooms, reconstituted in hot water and cut into thin strips

4 ounces water chestnuts, roughly chopped

4 celery stalks, thinly sliced

32 ounces cauliflower rice (approximately 4 cups)

1 tablespoon coconut aminos

¼ teaspoon powdered mustard

¼ teaspoon cayenne pepper (optional)

2 omega-3 or pastured eggs or VeganEggs, whisked (optional)

1. Heat the sesame oil in a large skillet or wok over medium-high heat.

2. Add the onion and ginger, and cook for 3 to 4 minutes, until the onions are translucent. Add the garlic and mushrooms, and cook an additional 2 to 3 minutes, until garlic is fragrant.

3. Add the water chestnuts and celery, and cook until vegetables soften (3 to 4 minutes).

4. Increase heat to high and add in the cauliflower rice. Cook for 3 to 4 more minutes, stirring frequently to ensure it doesn't burn.

5. Add 1 tablespoon of the coconut aminos, then add the mustard powder and cayenne, if using.

6. Continue cooking on high heat, stirring frequently, until the cauliflower is tender but not mushy.

7. If using eggs, make a well in the cauliflower rice and pour in the whisked eggs. Once they start to cook, stir them into the cauliflower rice. When the eggs have set, remove from heat and serve.

Sweet Potato Spaghetti and Meatballs

Spaghetti and meatballs are a weeknight classic for a reason, and you don't have to give them up on the Plant Paradox plan! The tender turkey meatballs are tossed in garlicky pesto sauce and served atop sweet potato noodles, which have become one of my favorite veggie noodles. They offer a hint of sweetness and fill you up.

SERVES 4

1 tablespoon salt

1 pound ground kosher turkey

½ brown onion, minced

1 clove garlic, crushed

1 omega-3 or pastured egg or VeganEgg

1 tablespoon Worcestershire sauce or coconut aminos

⅓ cup cassava flour

1 large sweet potato (about 1 pound), peeled and spiralized*

1 tablespoon extra-virgin olive oil

4 cups baby spinach

1 cup vegetable broth

1 cup Classic Basil Pesto (page 258)

FOR A VEGETARIAN ALTERNATIVE: *Sauté one package of Quorn grounds in olive oil, then mix with pesto, spinach, and noodles.*

1. Bring a large pot of water to a boil with the tablespoon of salt.

2. Meanwhile, mix the turkey, onion, garlic, egg or VeganEgg, Worcestershire sauce or coconut aminos, and cassava flour. Mixture should be thick enough to form cohesive meatballs. If they aren't, add additional cassava flour, half a teaspoon at a time.

3. Shape the meat mixture into small balls, about 2 tablespoons each. Refrigerate for 15 minutes.

4. When the water has reached a rolling boil, add the sweet potato noodles. Cook for 5 minutes, until tender, then remove from water and set aside.

5. Heat a large skillet over medium heat. Add the olive oil, and cook meatballs, turning occasionally, until golden brown on all sides.

6. Add the spinach and vegetable broth, turn heat to low, and cover pan. Cook for an additional 10 minutes, until the meatballs are cooked through and spinach is wilted.

7. Add the "noodles" and toss. Remove from heat, and gently fold in pesto before serving.

* If you don't have a spiralizer, cut noodles into thin strips with a very sharp knife, mandolin, or vegetable peeler.

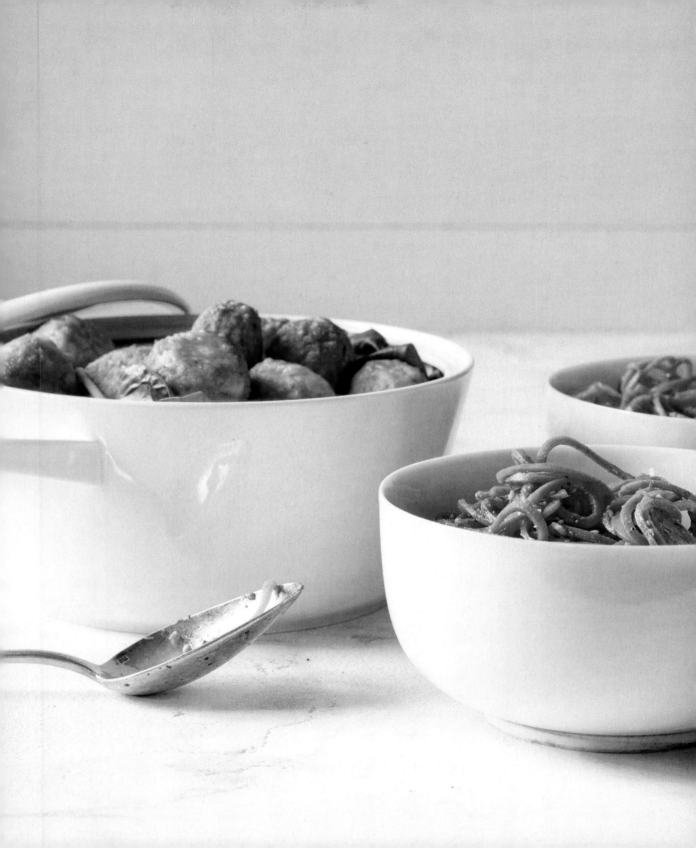

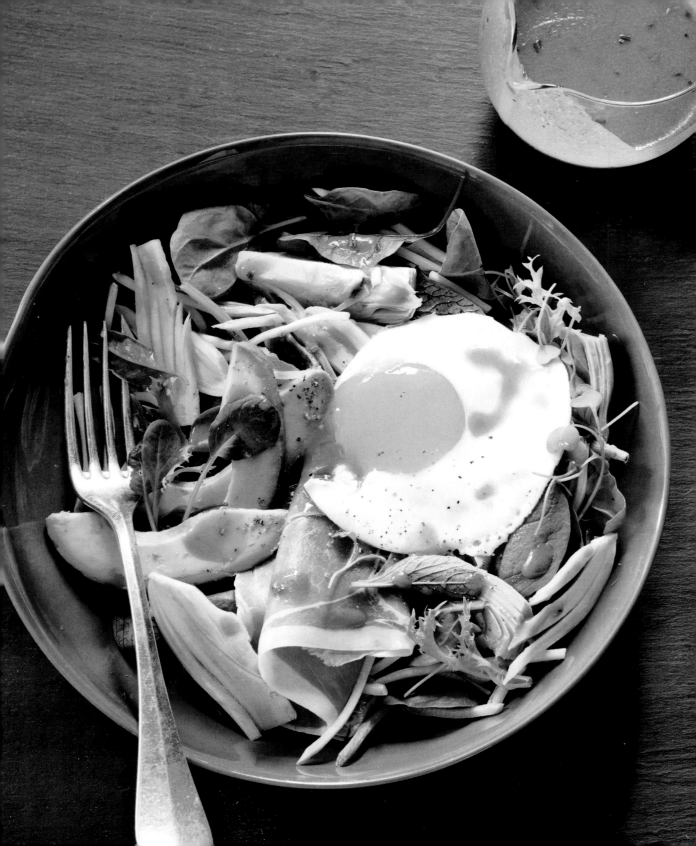

Greens with Eggs and Ham

Do you like greens, eggs, and ham? I sure do . . . especially when tossed with a tangy dressing! This lively take on a salad strikes just the right balance of filling and light—perfect for busy days.

SERVES 1

¼ cup Classic Balsamic Vinaigrette (page 260)

2 cups mixed baby greens

½ cup thinly sliced fennel

1 cup broccoli slaw

1 cup diced artichoke hearts (frozen and thawed)

½ avocado, cubed

1 tablespoon extra-virgin olive oil

2 omega-3 or pastured eggs or the other half of the avocado

2 ounces prosciutto, diced (optional)

1. In a large bowl, toss the vinaigrette with the greens, fennel, slaw, and artichoke hearts until well combined.

2. Add the avocado cubes and toss gently to coat. Set aside.

3. Heat the olive oil in a small skillet over medium heat. Add the eggs and cook until overeasy, then set aside.

4. Transfer the greens to a serving bowl, and top with prosciutto, if using, and eggs.

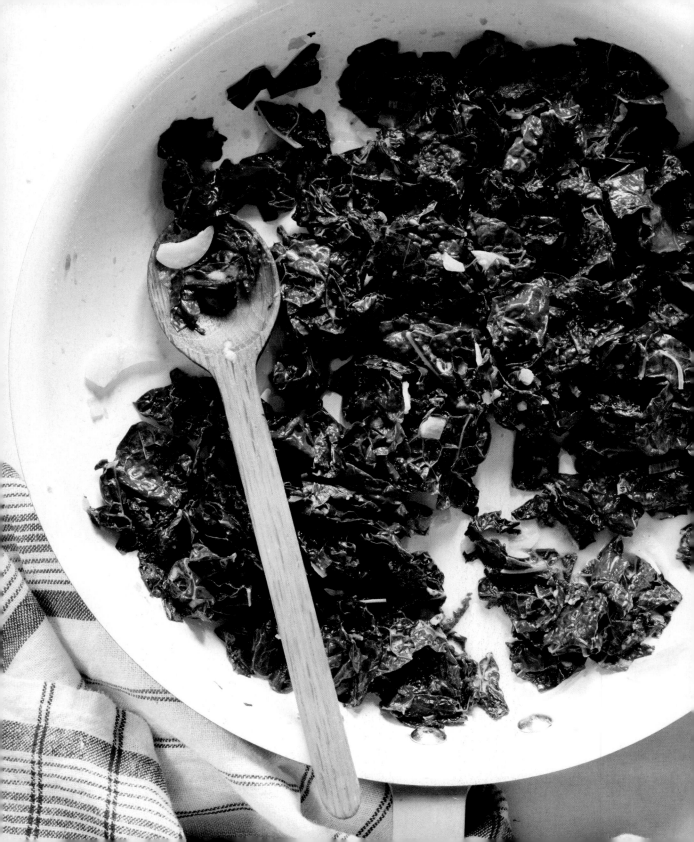

chapter ten

Vegetables and Sides

CRISPY BRUSSELS SPROUTS WITH BALSAMIC AND DATES

DR. G'S LECTIN-LIGHT CAPRESE SALAD

HERB-ROASTED RADISHES

PERFECT ROAST VEGGIES

THANKSGIVING MILLET STUFFING

WILD RICE SALAD

SPICED CARROT AND BROCCOLI SLAW

PROSCIUTTO-BRAISED CABBAGE

RALPH'S ROASTED CAULIFLOWER

SPICY SWEET POTATO FRITTERS

QUICK-PICKLED VEGETABLES

SWEET AND SOUR CABBAGE AND KALE SLAW

SORGHUM AND BEAN SALAD

TANGY COCONUT GREENS

SWEET POTATO FRIES WITH BLUE CHEESE DIP

Crispy Brussels Sprouts with Balsamic and Dates

This recipe comes courtesy of Irina Skoeries, founder of Catalyst Cuisine and dear friend of ours. If you're on Phase 1 or 2, feel free to skip the dates—these tender-yet-crispy Brussels sprouts are still great without them.

SERVES 4

1 pound Brussels sprouts, stems removed, cut in half

½ cup avocado oil or olive oil

2 teaspoons iodized sea salt, divided

1 tablespoon balsamic reduction*

½ cup pitted dates, finely chopped

Juice of ½ lemon

½ cup slivered toasted almonds

1. Preheat the oven to 350°F.

2. Toss the halved Brussels sprouts in the oil and spread in single layer on baking sheet. Sprinkle with salt.

3. Bake for 20 to 30 minutes, until the Brussels sprouts are golden, and a bit crunchy on the outside and soft on the inside.

4. Let the sprouts cool. While they are still warm, add the balsamic reduction, salt, chopped dates, lemon juice, and toasted almonds.

5. Mix well and serve warm.

To make balsamic reduction, simply pour a half cup of balsamic vinegar into a small pan, cook over medium heat until syrupy, then keep in the refrigerator until needed.

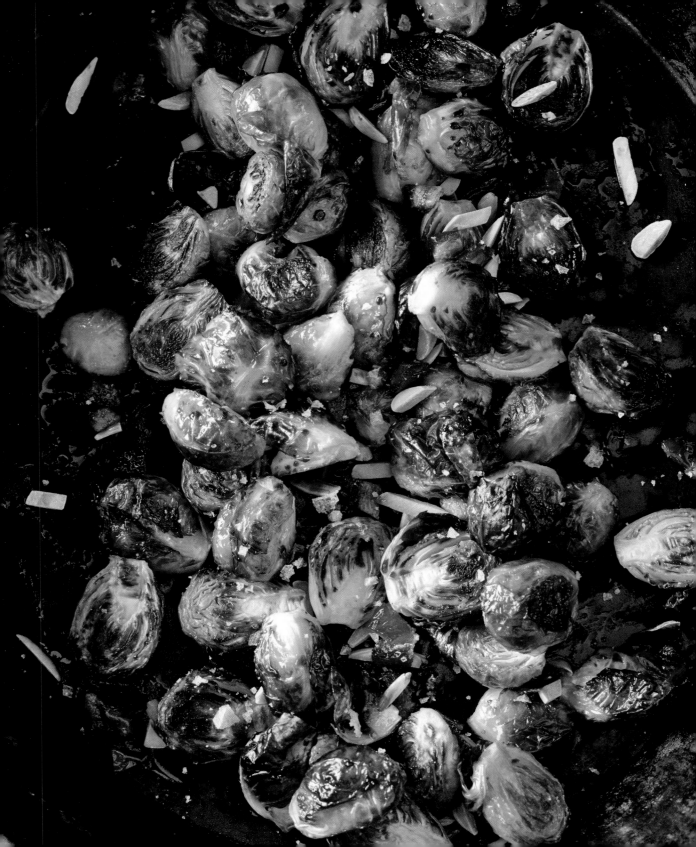

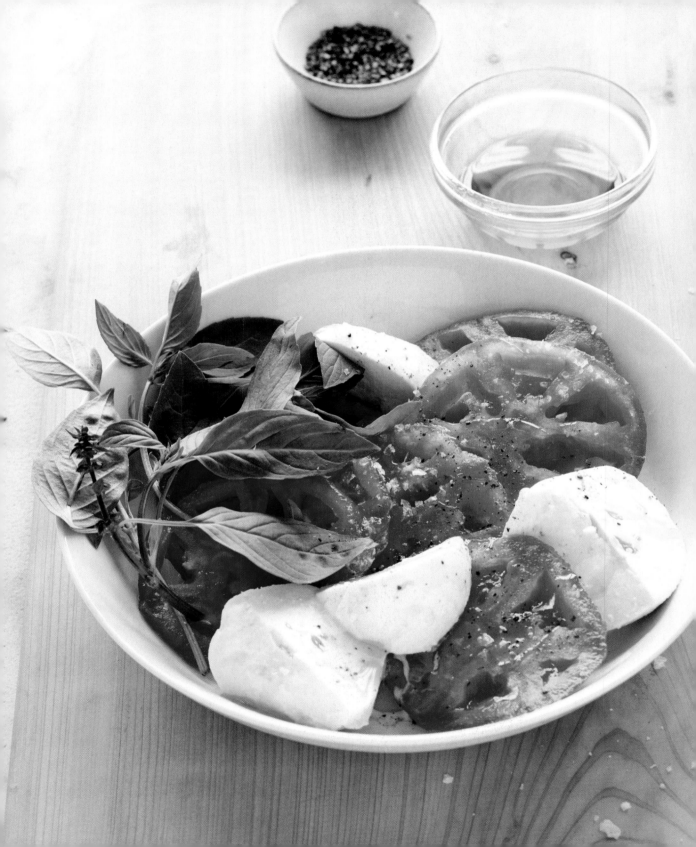

Dr. G's Lectin-Light Caprese Salad

Caprese salad is actually one of the dishes my patients tell me they miss the most on the Plant Paradox plan, especially in the summer months, when fresh tomatoes can be found in abundance. Good news! If you're on Phase 3 of the Plant Paradox program and you want to enjoy a tomato-rich Caprese salad, you can. Just peel and seed the tomatoes and dig right in!

SERVES 4

3 large tomatoes

2 cups salad greens (for serving)

¼ cup extra-virgin olive oil

2 tablespoons Classic Basil Pesto (page 258)

1 cup basil leaves

8 ounces buffalo mozzarella

¼ cup balsamic vinegar

½ teaspoon iodized sea salt

1. First, prepare the tomatoes: peel them with a serrated vegetable peeler, then cut them in half. Carefully scoop out the seeds and pulp of the tomatoes with a spoon, then slice with a serrated knife.

2. Place the greens in a large salad bowl and toss with the olive oil and pesto.

3. Arrange the tomatoes, basil leaves, and mozzarella on top of the greens.

4. Drizzle with balsamic vinegar and sea salt, and serve.

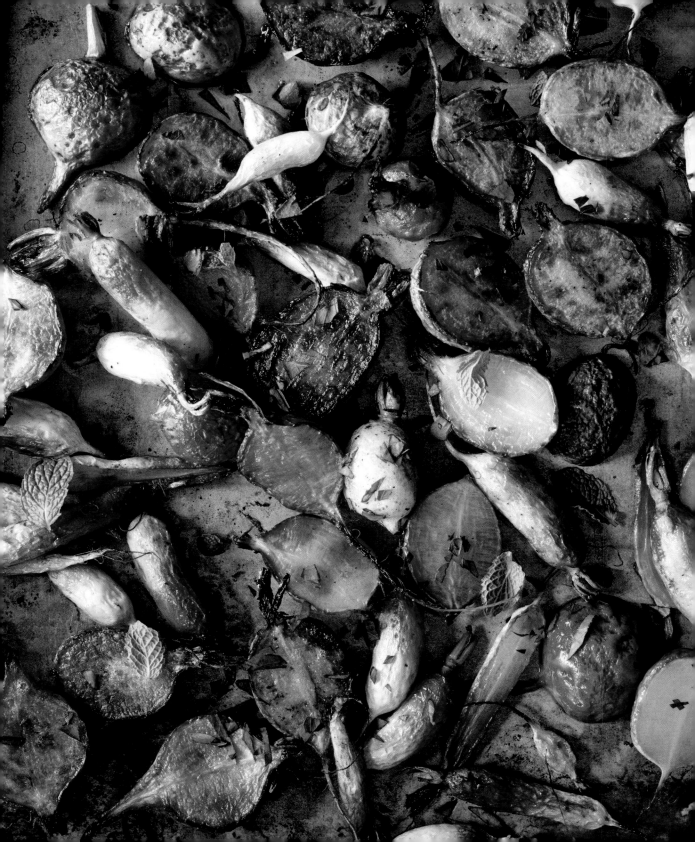

Herb-Roasted Radishes

Roasted potatoes are a classic side dish but, as we know, potatoes are part of the nightshade family and should be avoided. Luckily, radishes roast beautifully—and when tossed with fresh herbs and a bit of butter or oil, they make a perfect substitute for potatoes.

SERVES 4

1½ pound radishes, stems trimmed, quartered

4 tablespoons French or Italian grass-fed butter (such as Trader Joe's Cultured French Butter, President, or Beurre D'Insigny), melted, or avocado oil

1 teaspoon iodized sea salt

¼ cup minced parsley

¼ cup minced mint

1. Preheat the oven to 425°F.

2. Toss the radishes with half the butter or oil.

3. Spread into a single layer on a sheet tray and sprinkle with salt.

4. Bake for 20 to 25 minutes, until tender.

5. While radishes are baking, heat the rest of the butter or oil over medium-high heat in a small skillet. When hot, add the herbs and remove from heat.

6. Remove the radishes from oven skillet, and toss with herb mixture, right on the sheet tray. Serve hot or at room temperature.

Perfect Roast Veggies

Roasting transforms any vegetable into a hearty and flavorful side dish. If you haven't yet mastered this deceptively simple skill, let me share with you my foolproof technique. The only variable is cooking time—some vegetables take a bit longer than others. Just refer to the handy chart here and you can't go wrong.

SERVES 4 TO 6

2 pounds of your favorite vegetables, cut into bite-size pieces

3 cloves garlic, thinly sliced

2 tablespoons minced fresh rosemary

Zest of 1 orange

1 teaspoon iodized sea salt

½ cup extra-virgin olive oil

1. Preheat the oven to 425°F.

2. Toss the veggies with the garlic, rosemary, orange zest, salt, and olive oil.

3. Roast until tender on the inside and golden brown on the edges (see chart for more specific cooking times).

4. To make them even more special, consider sprinkling your freshly roasted veggies with a little balsamic vinegar or balsamic reduction.

VEGETABLE	COOK TIME	NOTES
ASPARAGUS	10 to 15 minutes	Roast whole (ends trimmed). Try with slivered almonds, or swap out the orange zest for lemon zest.
BROCCOLI	20 to 25 minutes	Cut florets into bite-size pieces and stems a little smaller. Definitely try the balsamic drizzle!
CAULIFLOWER	30 to 35 minutes	Cut into bite-size florets before roasting—try sprinkling with a little grated Parmigiano-Reggiano cheese before serving.
FENNEL	20 to 25 minutes	Slice into quarter-inch slices before roasting. Great with fish!
GREENS	10 to 15 minutes	Remove tough stems from all greens except chard (those are delicious). And keep a close eye on greens, as they can go from perfect to burnt quickly.
MUSHROOMS	20 to 25 minutes	Halve or quarter small mushrooms; cut large ones, like portabellas, into slices. Swap rosemary for thyme.
OKRA	15 to 20 minutes	Cut in half lengthwise and roast cut-side up to reduce sliminess.

VEGETABLE	COOK TIME	NOTES
ONIONS	25 to 35 minutes	Roast medium to large onions quartered, and smaller onions (or shallots) whole.
SWEET POTATOES	30 to 35 minutes	Cut into bite-size chunks (one quarter or eighth of a potato, depending on how small they are).

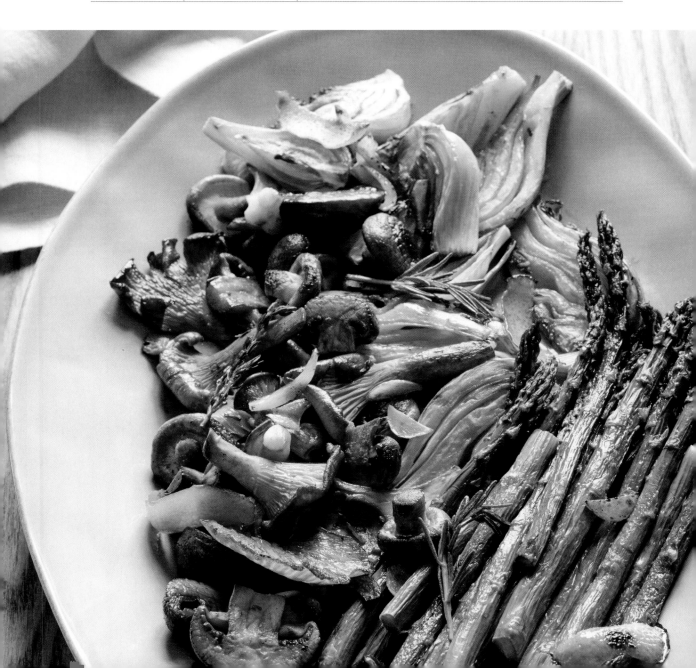

Thanksgiving Millet Stuffing

We came up with this recipe for a Thanksgiving-themed episode on my YouTube channel, but it's become a favorite of mine year-round. After all, when people think "stuffing," it's more about the savory flavors—particularly onion and sage—than the bread, so swapping out the starch lets everyone enjoy their favorite side dish, guilt free.

SERVES 4 TO 6

¼ cup plus 1 tablespoon French or Italian grass-fed butter (such as Trader Joe's Cultured French Butter, President, or Beurre D'Insigny) or olive oil spray for pan

3 cups cooked millet (prepared according to package instructions)

2 yellow onions, finely diced

3 carrots, finely diced

3 celery stalks, finely diced

5 cloves garlic, minced

1½ tablespoons minced fresh sage

1 tablespoon minced fresh parsley

2 tablespoons dried poultry seasoning (no salt added)

1 pound mushrooms, finely diced

1 teaspoon minced fresh thyme

½ teaspoon sea salt

½ teaspoon ground black pepper

1. Preheat the oven to 350°F. Butter your favorite 9 × 13-inch casserole dish with 1 tablespoon butter, or spray it with 1 tablespoon olive oil, and set aside.

2. Add the cooked millet to a large mixing bowl and set aside.

3. In a large skillet or wok, heat half the butter or oil over medium-high heat. Add the carrots, celery, and onions, and cook until tender, stirring regularly.

4. Add the garlic, sage, parsley, and poultry seasoning, and cook for 2 to 3 minutes more, until mixture is very fragrant. Add to bowl with millet.

5. Heat the rest of the oil or butter in the same skillet, and add the mushrooms and thyme.

6. Cook until the mushrooms are golden brown and tender, then add to the millet mixture.

7. Stir in the stuffing mixture to combine. Season with salt and pepper.

8. Add the stuffing to the baking dish, and bake for 25 to 35 minutes, until stuffing is hot all the way through, and the top is golden brown.

Wild Rice Salad

This savory wild rice salad is a beautifully balanced side dish that's perfect for anyone in Phase 3 of the Plant Paradox program. And since the wild rice is pressure-cooked, you don't have to worry about the lectins—or the long cook time of a traditionally-prepared rice dish.

SERVES 4

¼ cup plus 1 tablespoon extra-virgin olive oil

1 onion, diced

2 cups wild rice

3 cups Vegetable Stock (page 265)

½ cup roasted pine nuts

6 green onions or scallions, chopped

8 ounces crumbled goat feta (optional)

Iodized sea salt and pepper, to taste

1. Pour 1 tablespoon olive oil into a pressure cooker, and heat on the stove over medium-high heat (or on the sauté setting of an electric pressure cooker).

2. Add the onion and cook until tender, then add the rice, and sauté an additional 2 to 3 minutes.

3. Add the broth and set the pressure cooker for rice. Cook for 30 minutes.

4. When finished, keep the lid on for 1 to 2 hours so the rice continues to cook in its own heat.

5. Add the remaining quarter cup of olive oil to the rice, then add the pine nuts, green onion or scallions, and feta, if using. Stir to combine.

6. Season with salt and pepper as needed. Serve warm or at room temperature.

Spiced Carrot and Broccoli Slaw

I've always loved coleslaw for its perfect balance of sweetness, crunch, and tang. This twist on classic slaw switches things up a little by adding Moroccan-inspired spices you don't usually associate with coleslaw.

SERVES 4 TO 6

2 cups broccoli slaw

1 cup shredded red cabbage

2 cups shredded carrots

1 cup pickled red onions (see Quick-Pickled Vegetables, page 208)

¼ cup extra-virgin olive oil

2 cloves garlic, minced

1 tablespoon minced ginger

½ teaspoon cinnamon

1 teaspoon paprika

½ teaspoon cumin

1 teaspoon turmeric

1 teaspoon iodized sea salt

2 cups coconut or goat's milk yogurt

1. In a large bowl, toss together the broccoli slaw, red cabbage, carrots, and pickled red onions.

2. In a small sauté pan over medium heat, heat the olive oil, garlic, and ginger until fragrant. Add the cinnamon, paprika, cumin, turmeric, and sea salt, and cook for an additional 30 seconds to 1 minute, until spices are toasted.

3. Remove from heat and whisk in yogurt. Toss yogurt mixture with the slaw, and serve at room temperature (or chilled).

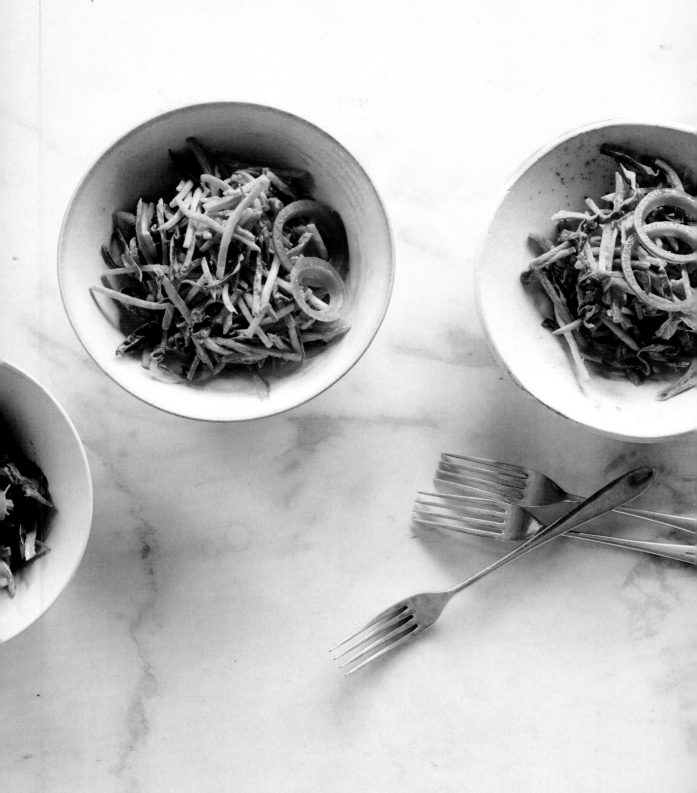

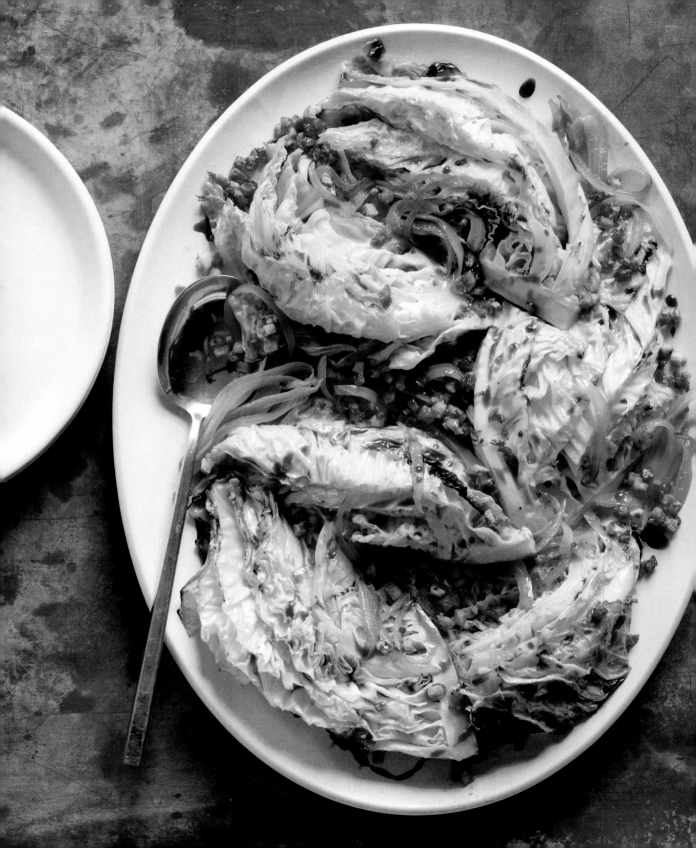

Prosciutto-Braised Cabbage

Cabbage and pork are a classic pairing, but most commercially available pork comes from animals fattened up with corn and grain. That's why I love to use Prosciutto di Parma in my dishes—this particular type of prosciutto is made in specific regions of Italy from heritage breeds of pigs raised according to the highest standards of care. The prosciutto in this dish breaks down to impossibly tender, melt-in-your-mouth bits that impart a delicious flavor. If you opt to go meat-free, you may want to increase the amount of salt called for in the directions below.

SERVES 4

2 tablespoons extra-virgin olive oil

1 1½-pound head of green cabbage, cut through the core into 6 wedges

½ cup chopped prosciutto, preferably Prosciutto di Parma (optional)

1 medium onion, thinly sliced

½ cup apple cider vinegar

1 cup Vegetable Stock (page 265)

1 teaspoon iodized sea salt

¼ cup pomegranate molasses

1. In a large, deep skillet, heat the olive oil until shimmering.

2. Add the cabbage wedges, cut-side down, and cook over medium heat until browned, 6 to 8 minutes, turning occasionally to prevent burning. Set aside.

3. Add the prosciutto and onion to the skillet, and cook over medium heat, stirring occasionally, until onions are tender and prosciutto is beginning to crisp.

4. Stir in the vinegar, and simmer over medium-high heat until reduced by half, about 3 minutes. Add the broth and salt and bring to a boil.

5. Return the cabbage wedges to the skillet, cover, and braise over medium-low heat, turning once, until tender, about 20 minutes.

6. Using a slotted spoon or spatula, transfer the cabbage to a platter and tent with foil until serving.

7. Serve drizzled with pomegranate molasses.

Ralph's Roasted Cauliflower

One night when my patients—and now friends—Ralph and Steve had us over for dinner, they served this interesting twist on a classic roasted cauliflower. It makes a great presentation, since you're serving it whole, rather than cut into florets. In fact, if you're ever cooking a meatless special-occasion meal, I'd suggest making this for your entrée.

SERVES 4 TO 5

¼ cup plus 3 tablespoons extra-virgin olive oil

1 head cauliflower, green leaves discarded

1 teaspoon iodized sea salt

1 tablespoon fresh lemon juice, or to taste

1 tablespoon drained small capers

1 teaspoon monk-fruit sweetener or 1 packet stevia

¼ teaspoon black pepper

¼ cup chopped fresh flat-leaf parsley (optional)

1. Put an oven rack in the middle position and preheat the oven to 450°F. Lightly oil a 9-inch pie plate or square baking dish.

2. Remove only the core from the cauliflower, leaving head intact, then place the cauliflower in the pie plate or baking dish, core-side down.

3. Drizzle 3 tablespoons olive oil over the top of cauliflower, and sprinkle with half a teaspoon salt, then place the pie plate or baking dish in the oven.

4. Bake until tender, 1 hour to 1 hour and 15 minutes (length of time varies by oven and size of cauliflower; I recommend you check tenderness periodically). Cauliflower should appear somewhat blackened. When done, transfer to a serving dish.

5. Whisk together the lemon juice, capers, monk-fruit sweetener or stevia, pepper, and the remaining half teaspoon salt in a small bowl, then whisk in the remaining quarter cup of oil.

6. Sprinkle the cauliflower with the parsley, if using, then drizzle with dressing.

Spicy Sweet Potato Fritters

These sweet and spicy fritters are packed with flavor and offer a satisfying crunch. They make a great side dish, starter, or even main course. Try serving them with my Blue Cheese Dip (page 215) or Caramelized Onion Dip (page 85).

SERVES 8 TO 10

5 cups peeled and spiralized sweet potatoes*

¼ cup tapioca flour

¼ cup almond flour

½ cup thinly sliced scallions

½ cup minced shallots

½ teaspoon cayenne pepper

1 or 2 pinches of cumin

2 omega-3 or pastured eggs or VeganEggs

1 to 2 cups coconut oil (for cooking)

1 teaspoon iodized sea salt

1. Add the sweet potatoes to a large bowl, and chop into 1- or 2-inch pieces with kitchen scissors.

2. Add the tapioca flour, almond flour, scallions, shallots, cayenne pepper, cumin, and eggs.

3. Mix together until the potatoes are well coated in flour and the mixture is holding together nicely.

4. Shape into small patties, about 4 inches in diameter.

5. Using a large skillet, heat 2 to 3 tablespoon of coconut oil over medium heat.

6. Once the oil is hot, place the patties in the skillet. Cook the patties until they are golden brown, about 4 to 6 minutes, then flip and cook the other sides for another 2 minutes. (For each additional batch, you may need to add more coconut oil to skillet.)

7. These are best when eaten right off the skillet, topped with sea salt.

If you don't have a spiralizer, you can cut potatoes into thin noodles with a vegetable peeler.

Quick-Pickled Vegetables

One of the best (and healthiest) ways to add flavor to a dish is by tossing in some chopped pickled veggies. But most commercially pickled veggies aren't part of the Plant Paradox program: either they're pickled in a sugar-and-salt brine, or they're cucumbers, with seeds and skins. This no-fuss quick pickle method couldn't be easier. Once you make your first batch of homemade pickles, you'll be hooked!

NUMBER OF SERVINGS VARIES

2 cups Plant Paradox–approved veggies, sliced into bite-size pieces (see guide below)

5 to 6 cloves garlic, sliced

¼ to ½ cup fresh herbs (see guide below)

1 cup red vinegar (see guide below), plus more if needed

2 tablespoon iodized sea salt

1 packet stevia

1. Pack veggies, garlic, and herbs into a clean quart-size jar, leaving a half inch of headspace (these are refrigerator pickles, so no need to fully sterilize your jar).

2. In a saucepan, heat the vinegar, salt, and stevia until boiling.

3. Carefully pour vinegar mixture into jar until it covers veggies (add more if needed).

4. Let cool to room temperature, then refrigerate until ready (see guide below).

5. Will keep up to 3 weeks, refrigerated.

VEGETABLE	HERBS	VINEGAR	MINIMUM WAIT TIME
BEETS	Orange zest, parsley	Red wine	3 hours
BROCCOLI STEMS	Lemon zest, parsley	Red wine	3 hours
DAIKON	Chives, mint	Rice wine	2 hours
CARROTS	Parsley, mint	White balsamic	2 hours
FENNEL	Dill, lemon zest	White balsamic	1 hour
GINGER	Chives	Rice wine	30 minutes
OKRA	Parsley, thyme	Apple cider	1 hour
ONIONS	Rosemary, thyme	Apple cider	1 hour
RADISHES	Thyme, parsley	Red wine	1½ hours

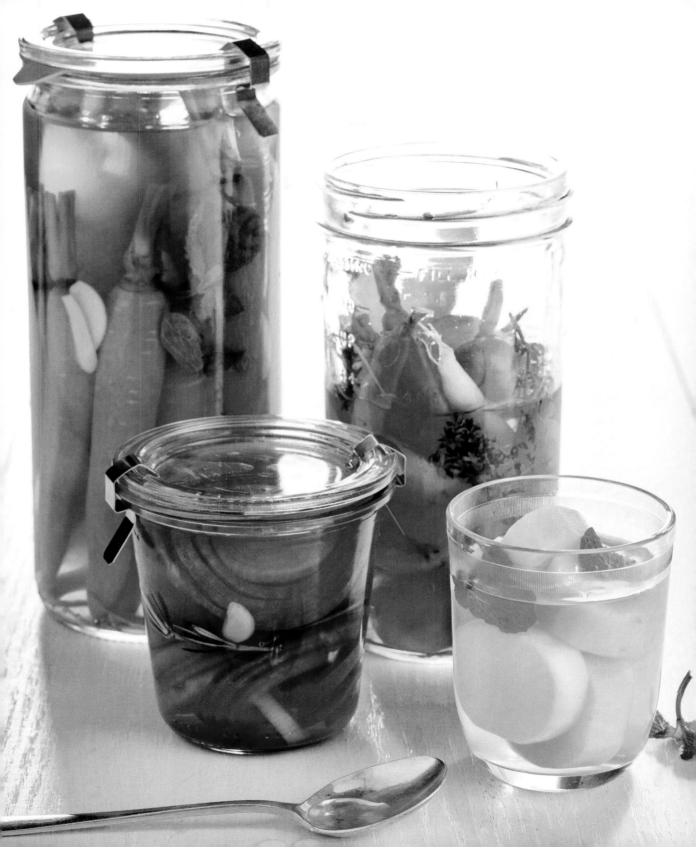

Sweet and Sour Cabbage and Kale Slaw

You might scan this ingredient list and think, Dried figs? I thought I was supposed to "give fruit the boot"? Yes, you are, but the thing about figs is that they're actually a flower, and they're incredibly high in gut-healthy fiber. Though if you're on Phase 1, I'd suggest skipping this recipe or omitting the figs.

SERVES 4

2 cups thinly sliced kale, ribs removed

½ teaspoon iodized sea salt

1 cup coconut yogurt

1 tablespoon Dijon mustard

Juice of 1 lemon

1 teaspoon garlic powder

½ teaspoon paprika

2 tablespoons pomegranate molasses or balsamic reduction

2 cups thinly sliced cabbage

1 red onion, thinly sliced

½ cup dried figs (no sugar added), diced

1. In a large bowl, massage the kale with salt until tender.

2. In a small bowl, combine the yogurt, Dijon mustard, lemon juice, garlic powder, paprika, and pomegranate molasses or balsamic reduction.

3. Add the dressing to the kale, along with the cabbage, onion, and figs, and toss to combine.

4. Serve chilled or at room temperature.

Sorghum and Bean Salad

This simple "grain" and bean salad offers plenty of fiber and protein, and can be served warm or cold. It travels well and makes a great side dish for a potluck or summer picnic. It's also a cinch to make—especially if you use Eden brand canned beans, which are pressure-cooked. Just rinse and they're ready to go!

SERVES 6 TO 8

1 16-ounce bag of sorghum

32 ounces (4 cups) water

3 cups pressure-cooked garbanzo beans (Eden Brand, drained, or homemade

4 celery stalks (leaves and all), sliced

1 red onion, diced

1 cup minced flat leaf parsley

2 cups minced cilantro

Juice of 6 limes

Zest of 2 limes

¼ cup extra-virgin olive oil

½ teaspoon cayenne pepper

Iodized sea salt, to taste

1. Place sorghum and water in your pressure cooker, and cook for approximately 25 minutes (until al dente).*

2. Release pressure from cooker, then drain and rinse sorghum in cold water.

3. Transfer sorghum to a large bowl, along with garbanzo beans, celery, red onion, parsley, and cliantro, and toss to combine.

4. Add lime juice, lime zest, olive oil, cayenne pepper, and a pinch of sea salt.

5. Mix well then taste. Add more salt as needed.

* If you don't have a pressure cooker, cook sorghum as you would rice (1 part sorghum, 3 parts water) until al dente—approximately 1 hour.

Tangy Coconut Greens

This delicious recipe was created by Jessica Murnane, author of the cookbook *One Part Plant* and creator of the food blog by the same name. While she uses kale here, she suggests that you can make this dish with any type of hearty, leafy green—Swiss chard, collard greens, or even bok choy. (If you use collards, just be sure to give them a little more time to cook down.)

SERVES 4

1 teaspoon coconut oil

1 shallot, minced

3 garlic cloves, minced

1½-inch knob of fresh ginger, peeled and minced

½ teaspoon iodized sea salt

2 bunches lancinato (dinosaur) kale, sliced into thin ribbons

1 cup canned full-fat coconut milk

1 tablespoon apple cider vinegar

1. In a large pan over medium heat, add coconut oil.

2. When the pan is hot and the coconut oil has melted, sauté the shallot until soft and translucent.

3. Stir in the garlic and ginger, and cook for another minute, until the ginger and garlic become fragrant. Add salt.

4. Add the kale. It will seem like too much kale at first, but keep going; it will wilt as it cooks and become just the right amount.

5. Toss the kale around the pan and coat it well with the shallot, garlic, and ginger mixture.

6. After the kale has wilted nicely and turned bright green, around 3 minutes, stir in the coconut milk. Let it simmer for a few minutes, stirring a couple times.

7. Add the apple cider vinegar. Heat for another minute or so. Salt to taste.

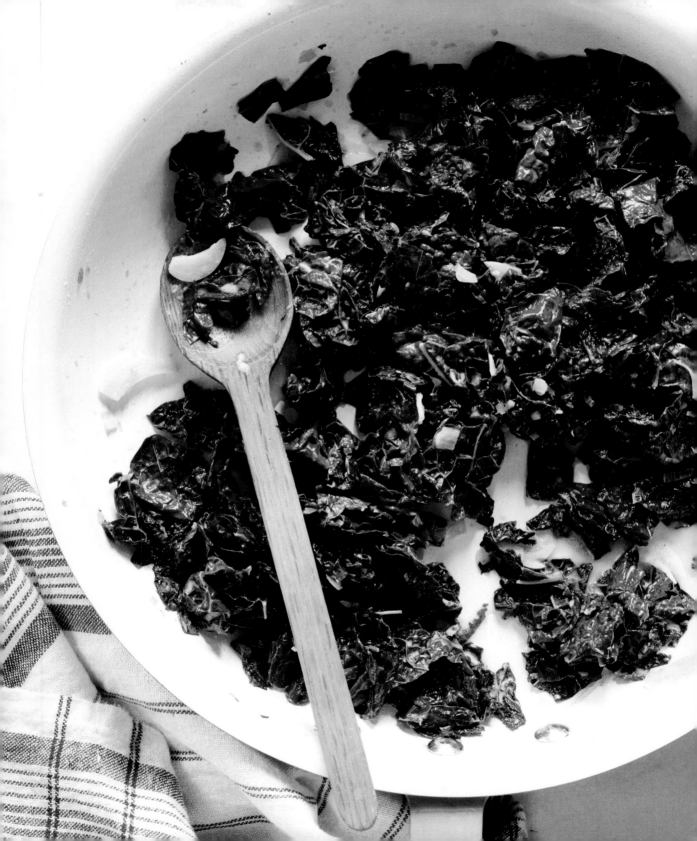

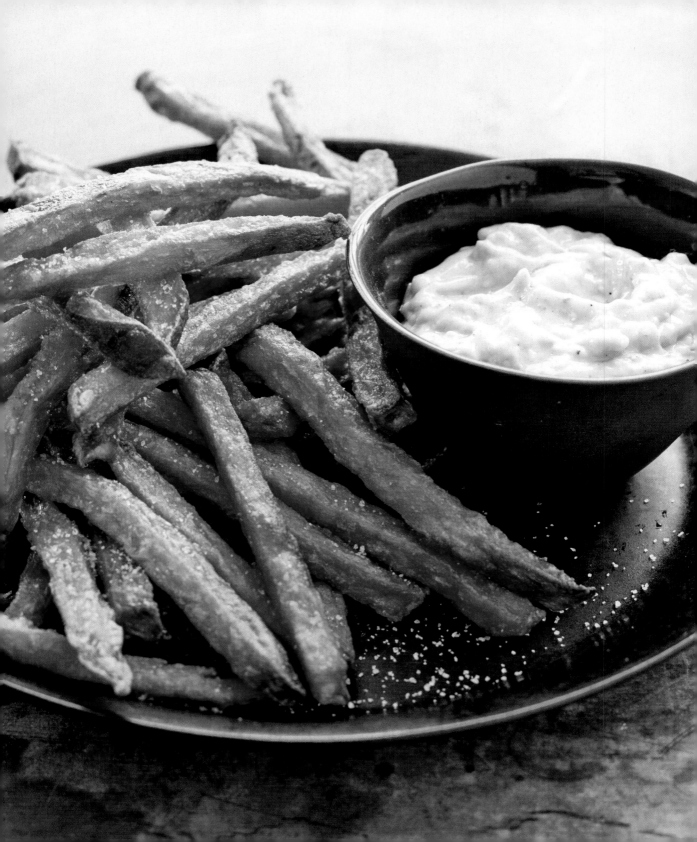

Sweet Potato Fries with Blue Cheese Dip

Who doesn't love a good french fry? This version, made with low-lectin sweet potatoes instead of lectin-rich white potatoes, is as delicious as it is good for your gut. If you want to create a "buffalo" twist, add a dash of Frank's Red Hot sauce to the blue cheese dip.

SERVES 4

FOR THE DIP

1 tablespoon extra-virgin olive oil or avocado oil

1 large garlic clove, minced

¼ teaspoon ground pepper

1¼ teaspoon champagne vinegar

½ cup crumbled Gorgonzola or raw cow's milk blue cheese*

FOR THE FRIES

¼ cup olive oil

1 teaspoon garlic powder

1 teaspoon sweet paprika

1 teaspoon iodized sea salt

½ teaspoon pepper

2 pounds sweet potato, peeled and cut into french fry-shape, or frozen organic sweet potato fries

1. First, make the dip: In a small bowl, combine all the ingredients and whisk until blue cheese breaks down and dip is creamy. (You can also do this in a high-speed blender.) Set aside.

2. Preheat the oven to 450°F. (Use a convection oven, if available.)

3. Put a large baking sheet inside oven during preheat—a hot tray means crispier fries.

4. In a large mixing bowl, combine the olive oil, garlic powder, paprika, salt, and pepper. Add sweet potatoes to the bowl, and toss so that ingredients cover them completely.

5. Remove the hot tray from oven and transfer the fries onto the tray. Spread in a single layer.

6. Return the tray to the oven and place on top rack. Cook sweet potatoes for 8 minutes, then flip.

7. Cook for another 15 to 17 minutes, tossing as needed, until the fries are crispy and golden brown.

Or 1 cup coconut yogurt, plus 1 tablespoon nutritional yeast.

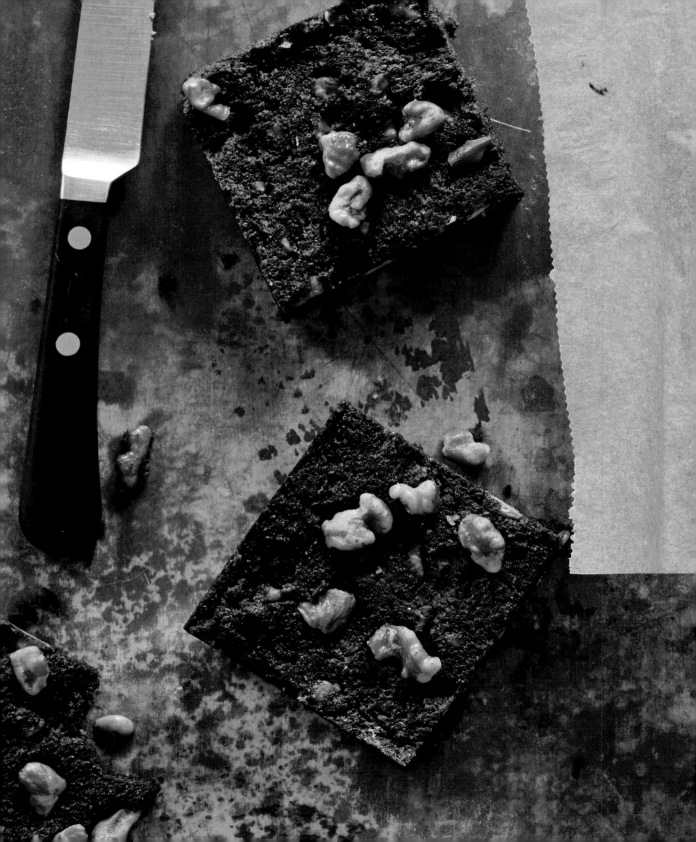

chapter eleven

Sweet Bites

ALMOND DELIGHT GRASSHOPPER ICE CREAM

PISTACHIO ICE CREAM

COCONUT OLIVE OIL ICE CREAM

LEMON POPPY COFFEE CAKE

CHOCOLATE CREAM PIE

CHOCOLATE MINT COOKIES

OLIVE OIL ROSEMARY CAKE

DRIED FIG "TRUFFLES"

FUNNEL CAKE WITH BLUEBERRY SAUCE

GINGER BROWNIE BITES

CINNAMON SWEET POTATO BLONDIES

PECAN PIE

PLANT PARADOX PIECRUST

Almond Delight Grasshopper Ice Cream

This sweet treat has all the flavor of a certain classic candy bar, but without the corn syrup and hydrogenated oils. With coconut cream, coconut flakes, toasted almonds, and bittersweet chocolate, this decadent dessert hits all the right notes. You won't taste the avocado, but it adds creaminess and richness—and a lovely pale green color!

MAKES 1 QUART

2 15-ounce cans unsweetened coconut cream

½ cup Swerve sweetener or 10 pitted dates (if you're on Phase 3)

½ teaspoon vanilla extract

1 ripe avocado

½ cup unsweetened coconut flakes

½ cup slivered toasted almonds

½ cup chopped bittersweet chocolate (at least 72 percent cacao)

1. Make sure the bowl of your ice cream machine is well-frozen.*

2. Heat the coconut cream in a large saucepan, along with the Swerve sweetener or dates and vanilla extract, and simmer on low until mixture is warmed through and sweetener, if using, is dissolved.

3. In a high-speed blender or a food processor fitted with an S-blade, blend together the avocado and the coconut cream mixture until smooth.

4. Chill the mixture at least 4 hours, or ideally overnight.

5. Freeze according to the instructions on your ice cream machine. When the ice cream is almost frozen, add in the coconut flakes, toasted almonds, and chocolate.

6. Eat at soft-serve consistency, or transfer it to an airtight container and freeze for 1 to 2 hours until ready to enjoy. Note: This ice cream gets pretty hard in the freezer after a few hours, so allow it to thaw until scoopable.

If you don't have an ice cream machine, follow steps 2 and 3. Then fold the coconut, almonds, and chocolate into the mixture and transfer to a shallow, covered, freezer-safe container. Freeze, stirring every 20 to 30 minutes, until ice cream consistency (you may need to stir more frequently the colder it gets).

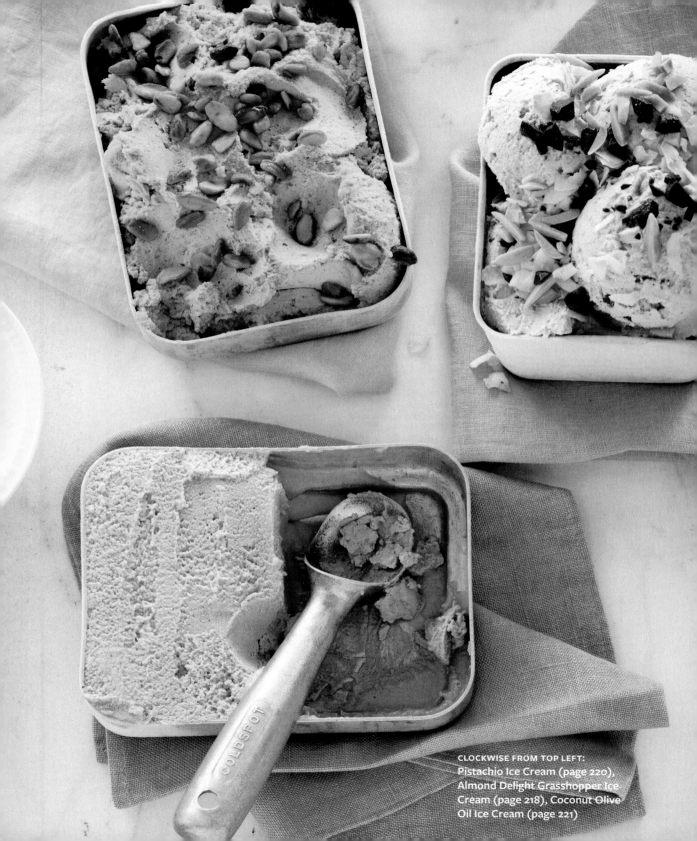

CLOCKWISE FROM TOP LEFT:
Pistachio Ice Cream (page 220),
Almond Delight Grasshopper Ice
Cream (page 218), Coconut Olive
Oil Ice Cream (page 221)

Pistachio Ice Cream

Any time I visit Italy, I find myself tempted by pistachio gelato—I absolutely love the flavor and the richness of it. So when it came time to develop recipes for this book, I wanted to include a Plant Paradox–approved version—and here it is! The deep pistachio flavor comes from roasted pistachios, and richness is added by coconut cream and avocado. Now, if only I could enjoy a scoop of this while strolling through the streets of Rome!

MAKES 1 GENEROUS PINT

2 cups coconut cream

½ cup Swerve (erythritol)

1 vanilla bean, split

1 cup roasted shelled pistachios (unsalted, if possible)

1 large avocado, skin and pit removed

¼ teaspoon iodized sea salt (unless using salted pistachios)

1. Heat the coconut cream, Swerve, and vanilla bean over low heat (keep it at a simmer, if possible), for about 5 to 10 minutes until Swerve dissolves

2. Add the pistachios and simmer on low for 20 to 30 minutes to infuse flavor.

3. Transfer mixture to a high-speed blender and blend until smooth.

4. Add the avocado and sea salt and blend until smooth.

5. Let chill in refrigerator until very cold, then freeze according to the manufacturer's instructions for your ice cream machine.*

6. Serve immediately at soft-serve consistency, or transfer to freezer to let set further. Note: Since this freezes pretty hard, let thaw a bit at room temperature before scooping.

If you don't have an ice cream machine, freeze in a loaf pan and stir every 20 to 30 minutes until set.

Coconut Olive Oil Ice Cream

Olive oil and rosemary meld together beautifully in both savory and sweet applications, and I love this classic pairing in ice cream. I went easy on the rosemary here, but feel free to add more if you prefer a more pronounced rosemary flavor.

SERVES 2 TO 4

1 can full-fat coconut milk or coconut cream (1⅔ cups)

⅓ cup yacón syrup or pureed dates

1 teaspoon diced fresh rosemary (optional)

3 omega-3 or pastured egg yolks, or 2 VeganEggs

⅔ cup very high quality extra-virgin olive oil

½ teaspoon vanilla extract

¼ teaspoon salt

* If you don't have an ice cream machine, follow steps 1 through 8, then transfer to a shallow covered freezer-safe container. Freeze, stirring every 20 to 30 minutes until ice cream consistency (you may need to stir more frequently the colder it gets).

** If the custard boils, the egg will curdle. If this happens, remove from heat immediately and pulse through a blender until smooth.

1. If using an ice cream machine, make sure the work bowl is chilled.*

2. Heat the coconut milk or cream, yacón syrup, and rosemary, if using, on medium-low heat, stirring very frequently, until hot and steaming, but just short of a simmer.

3. Separate the eggs and place the yolks in a heat-safe container. (A Pyrex bowl cup works well.)

4. Temper the egg yolks by adding a ladle full of hot milk to the yolks while stirring to prevent scrambling.

5. Add the tempered yolks to the saucepot, again stirring constantly.

6. Heat the mixture on medium-low, stirring constantly and never letting it simmer, until the custard thickens, about 6 to 8 minutes.**

7. Remove from heat and pour into a bowl or measuring cup to cool.

8. Transfer to blender, and add the rest of the ingredients. Blend until fully combined, then transfer to the refrigerator to chill.

9. When cold, transfer the chilled custard in your ice cream maker and freeze according to your manufacturer's instructions.

10. Serve at soft-serve consistency, or freeze for 1 to 4 hours to harden a little more before serving.

Lemon Poppy Coffee Cake

Yes, you can have your cake and eat it too! This delectable lemon-and-vanilla-scented cake is completely lectin-free, made from almond and coconut flour. This recipe produces a loaf-style cake, but you can double it and make it in a Bundt pan (as pictured) if you'd prefer something a little more elegant to serve guests.

SERVES 8

olive oil spray

1½ cups almond flour

¼ cup coconut flour

½ teaspoon salt

1 teaspoon baking soda

3 omega-3 or pastured eggs or VeganEggs

½ cup Swerve (erythritol)

¼ cup avocado oil

Juice of 3 lemons

Zest of 2 lemons

¼ cup unsweetened coconut milk

1 teaspoon vanilla extract

2 tablespoons poppy seeds

1. Spray a 9 × 5-inch loaf pan with olive oil and line it with parchment paper. Preheat the oven to 350°F.

2. In a large bowl, whisk together the almond flour, coconut flour, salt, and baking soda.

3. In a small bowl, combine the eggs, Swerve, avocado oil, lemon juice, lemon zest, coconut milk, and vanilla extract.

4. Whisk the wet ingredients into the dry ingredients until well combined.

5. Fold in the poppy seeds, then transfer dough to prepared loaf pan.

6. Bake for 35 to 40 minutes, or until a toothpick inserted into the middle of the loaf comes out clean.

7. Let cool for a few minutes before running a knife around the edge of the pan to help remove the loaf. Serve while still warm, or at room temperature.

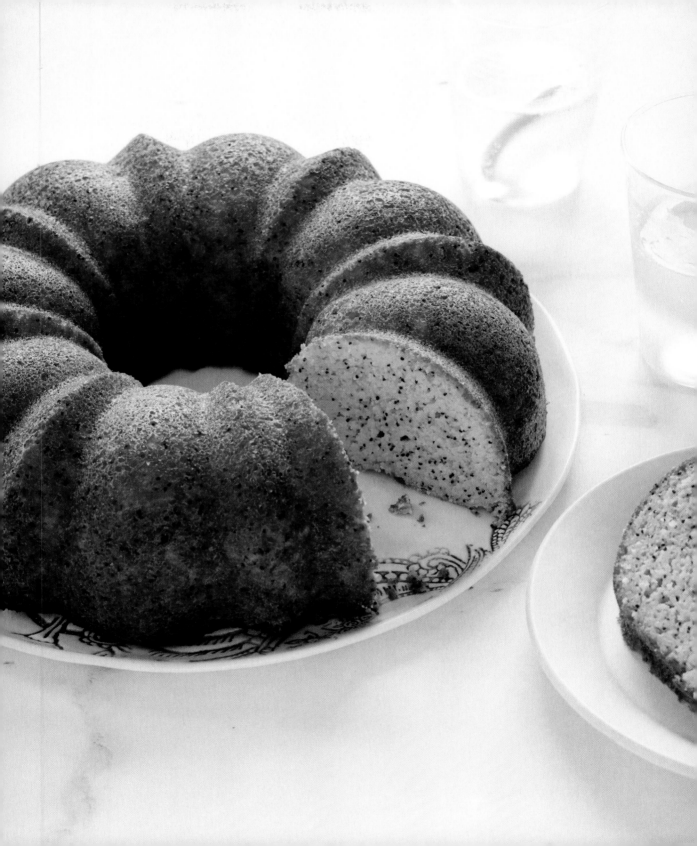

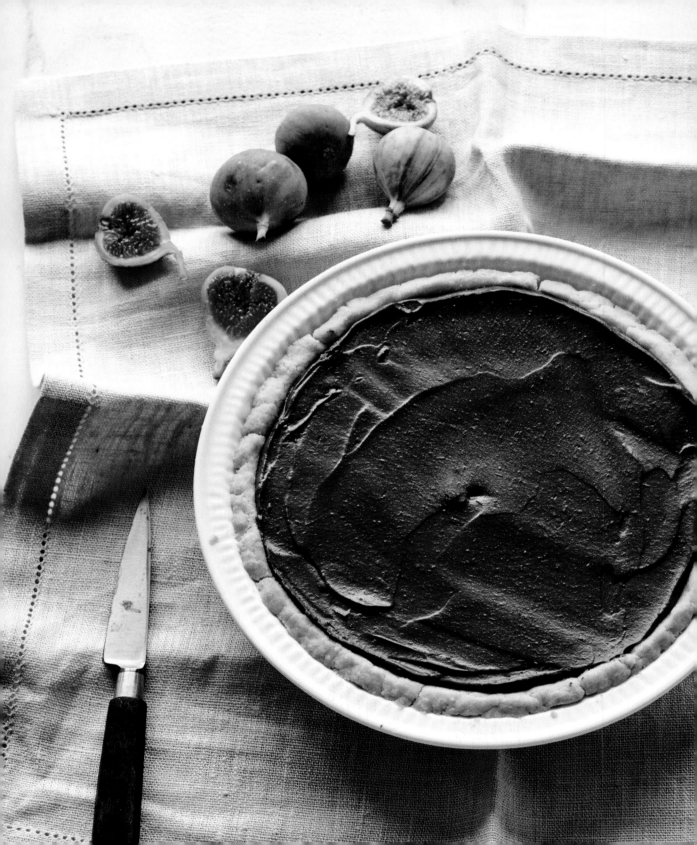

Chocolate Cream Pie

This recipe is inspired by a French silk pie I used to order at a local bakery. It was irresistible: a chocolatey and velvety smooth filling, complemented by a crispy shortbread crust. This Plant Paradox–approved version is just as satisfying, but a lot lighter. Make sure to let it set in the refrigerator for several hours so that when you cut into it, you get a beautiful slice!

SERVES 8

1 Plant Paradox Piecrust, baked (page 238)

½ cup coconut cream

⅔ cup granulated Swerve (erythritol)

2 ounces bittersweet chocolate (72 percent cacao or higher)

3 large ripe avocados, peeled and pitted

½ cup high-quality unsweetened cocoa powder

2 teaspoons pure vanilla extract

¼ teaspoon salt

Fresh, in-season fruit for serving (I suggest figs or berries)

1. Heat the coconut cream, Swerve, and chocolate in a small saucepan, stirring frequently until chocolate is melted and Swerve has dissolved. Set aside.

2. In a high-speed blender or a food processor fitted with an S-blade, blend the avocado, coconut cream mixture, cocoa powder, vanilla extract, and salt until smooth.

3. Transfer to prepared pie crust, making sure to smooth the mixture neatly on top.

4. Wrap well and refrigerate for at least 2 hours, or up to 2 days, before serving.

5. Let it come to room temperature before slicing, or cut it with a hot knife to melt through the chocolate with ease, and serve with fresh fruit. Store leftovers in the refrigerator, but allow pie to come to room temperature before serving.

Chocolate Mint Cookies

There's a reason chocolate and mint are a classic pairing—I can't think of two flavors that go better together. These easy-to-make-cookies come together quickly and make a great, simple weeknight dessert.

MAKES 12 LARGE OR 18 SMALL COOKIES

1 cup creamy almond butter

⅔ cup confectioner's Swerve (erythritol)

2 tablespoons non-Dutched cocoa powder

2 tablespoons blanched almond meal

1 tablespoon coconut flour

2 tablespoons water

2 large omega-3 or pastured eggs or VeganEggs

2 tablespoons melted, salted butter or coconut oil

1½ teaspoons pure peppermint extract

1 teaspoon baking soda

¼ cup chopped bittersweet chocolate

1. Preheat the oven to 350°F. Line a rimmed baking sheet with a silicone baking mat (a Silpat) or parchment paper.

2. In a large mixing bowl, combine the almond butter, erythritol, cocoa powder, almond meal, coconut flour, water, eggs, butter or oil, peppermint extract, and baking soda.

3. Using a stand mixer fitted with the paddle attachment, or a whisk and some serious arm strength, mix until all ingredients are well combined.

4. Fold in chopped chocolate.

5. Form the cookie dough into 2-inch balls to produce 12 cookies, or a bit smaller to make 18 cookies.

6. Place the cookie-dough balls on the prepared baking sheet, leaving room for them to spread.

7. Bake for 10 to 12 minutes. Allow cookies to cool before eating. Store any extra in an airtight container for 3 to 4 days.

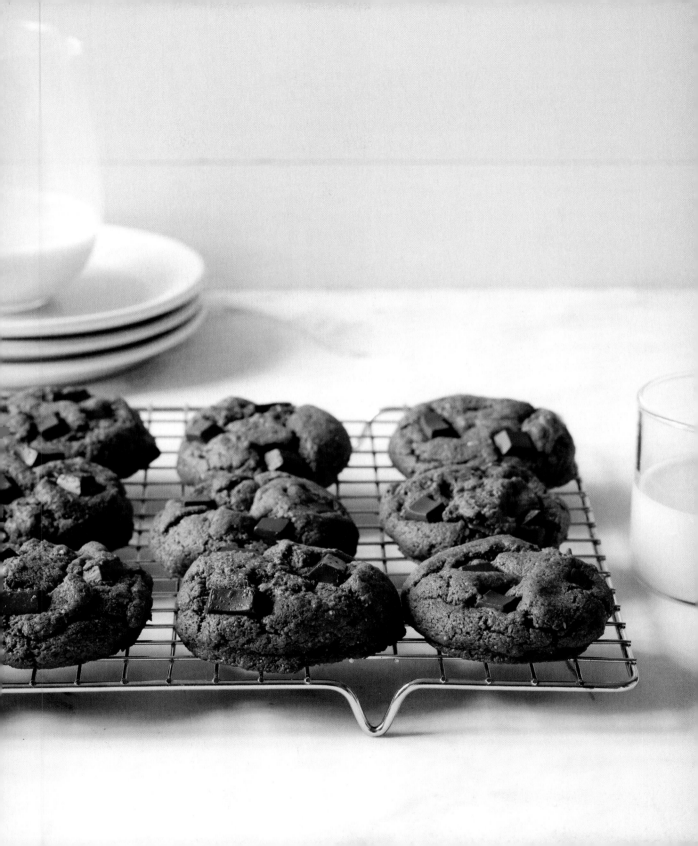

Olive Oil Rosemary Cake

This cake came from our recipe contest first-place winner, Nicola Moores. We were truly wowed by the flavor of the cake and the care she put into the recipe. Because I love the combination of orange and rosemary, we made one tweak and added a little orange zest to the batter, but you can omit this if you prefer. This dessert is a true stunner and sure to satisfy even the most discerning critics!

SERVES 8 TO 12

olive oil spray

1½ cups blanched almond flour

Zest of 1 orange

2 tablespoons rosemary leaves, roughly chopped

1 cup xylitol

2 teaspoon baking powder

Zest of 1 lemon

Juice of 1 lemon

⅔ cup extra-virgin olive oil

4 eggs, beaten

FOR THE SYRUP

½ cup water

Juice of 2 lemons

4 tablespoons xylitol

2 sprigs of rosemary

TO GARNISH

Rosemary sprigs

Goat's milk yogurt

1. Grease an 8-inch cake tin with olive oil. (Ideally, use a springform pan.)

2. In a food processor fitted with an S-blade, pulse the almond flour, orange zest, and rosemary until they're as fine as possible.

3. Transfer to a mixing bowl and stir in the xylitol, baking powder, and lemon zest. Add the lemon juice, olive oil, and eggs and mix until combined.

4. Pour the batter into prepared cake pan, then put into a cold oven. Turn the oven to 350°F. and bake for approximately 25 to 30 minutes, or until a skewer inserted into the center of the cake comes out clean.

5. Leave in the tin for 5 to 10 minutes to cool.

6. While the cake is cooling, make the syrup. Gently heat all of the ingredients in a small saucepan over medium heat until the xylitol has dissolved.

7. Bring to a gentle boil for 5 minutes, allowing the rosemary to infuse. Remove rosemary sprigs.

8. Using a bamboo skewer or the end of a meat thermometer, pierce holes all over the cake. Pour the syrup over the cake while still warm.

9. Once cooled, serve garnished with rosemary sprigs and a dollop of goat's milk yogurt. Store leftovers in an airtight container at room temperature for 3 to 4 days.

Dried Fig "Truffles"

If you've got dried figs, you can make chocolate "truffles" in no time. It takes a little practice to get these just right, as dried figs are delicate and can break easily. I suggest having a few extras on hand for trial and error if you're making them for guests. But rest assured, even the ugly ones will taste delicious!

MAKES 12

12 whole dried unsweetened figs

1 cup boiling water

1 cup coconut cream

Zest of 1 orange

1 tablespoon chopped rosemary

1 cup chopped bittersweet chocolate, at least 72 percent cacao

1. Reconstitute the figs by letting them soak in boiling water until pliable, about 20 minutes.

2. Pat figs dry with a kitchen towel, and set aside.

3. Heat the coconut cream, orange zest, and rosemary in a small saucepan until simmering.

4. Reduce the heat to very low, and whisk in chocolate until melted.

5. Cool the chocolate mixture to room temperature, and transfer to a pastry bag fitted with a round tip.

6. Fill the figs with chocolate cream from the bottom (figs will have a small hole in the bottoms—perfect for stuffing) until full.

7. Let the figs set before serving—this will take 6 to 8 hours at room temperature, or 2 to 4 hours in the refrigerator. (Let them come to room temperature before serving.)

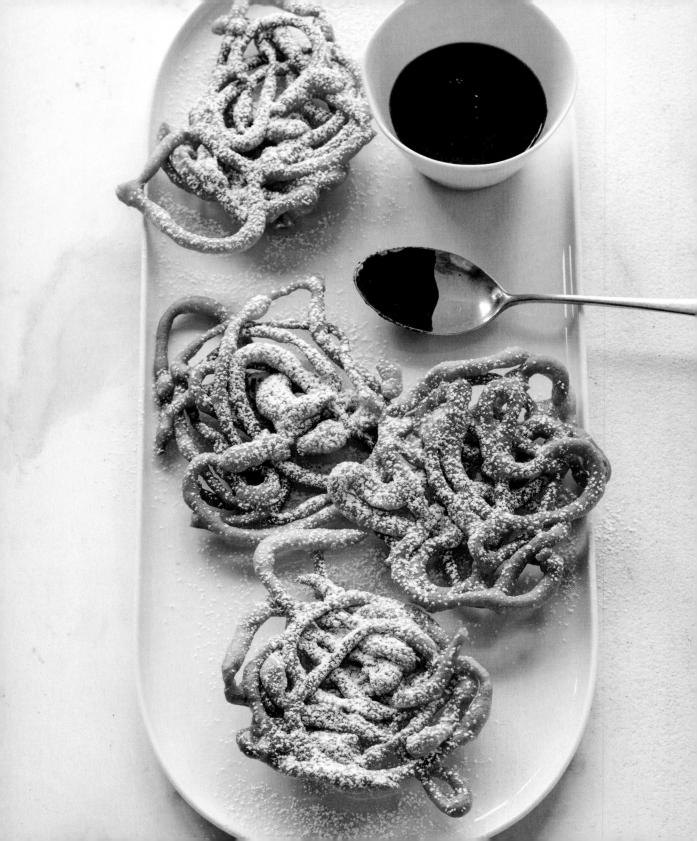

Funnel Cake with Blueberry Sauce

These funnel cakes are best served piping hot—like most fried foods, they get soggy when they sit for too long. If you're not on Phase 3, or blueberries aren't in season, skip the sauce and try them with a sprinkling of confectioner's Swerve or a drizzle of melted bittersweet chocolate!

SERVES 4

FOR THE SAUCE

2 cups wild blueberries (frozen okay)

1 teaspoon coconut oil

Zest of 1 lemon

Juice of 1 lemon

½ teaspoon cinnamon

8 to 10 drops stevia

FOR THE FUNNEL CAKES

1 cup tapioca flour

2 pastured or omega-3 eggs or VeganEggs

2 tablespoon yacón syrup or 1 tablespoon Swerve (erythritol)

2 tablespoon avocado oil

Pinch of iodized sea salt

Avocado oil for frying

1. First, make the blueberry sauce: In a small saucepan, combine all the ingredients, and cook over low heat until blueberries release their juices, about 5 minutes.

2. Transfer the blueberry sauce to a blender and pulse in blender until semi-smooth. Set aside until needed.

3. Combine the tapioca flour, eggs, yacón syrup or Swerve, avocado oil, and pinch of salt in a bowl, stirring until smooth. Set aside.

4. Pour about 1 inch of avocado oil into a small saucepan. Heat over medium heat until oil shimmers (you want this oil to reach about 350°F). Spoon the batter into a sandwich bag or pastry bag. Once the oil is shimmering (hot enough to fry), cut the tip of the sandwich bag, if using.

5. Now quickly drizzle the batter into the hot oil, overlapping to make that classic funnel cake squiggle.

6. Allow the underside to brown, around 1 minute, then, using a flat slotted spoon, flip the funnel cake over to brown the other side.

7. Remove from the oil and place on a towel-lined plate.

8. Serve hot, drizzled with blueberry sauce.

Ginger Brownie Bites

These rich, fudgy little bites are just the thing to finish off a special meal. I love the flavor of ginger, especially when combined with chocolate, but if you're not a fan you can omit it for a more traditional brownie taste. Either way, these treats are sure to satisfy when you need just a little bite of something sweet.

SERVES 12 TO 16

1 cup over 80 percent cacao chocolate, cut into small pieces

¼ cup French or Italian butter, softened, or coconut oil

¾ cup monk-fruit sweetener (use a spice grinder to make into powder) or ⅓ cup Swerve (erythritol)

½ teaspoon iodized sea salt

3 teaspoons grated fresh ginger

1 teaspoon almond extract

2 large omega-3 or pastured eggs or VeganEggs

⅔ cup blanched almond flour

⅓ cup tapioca starch

1 cup chopped toasted walnuts or toasted slivered almonds (optional)

1. Preheat the oven to 325°F. and line an 8 × 8-inch baking pan with parchment paper.

2. In a double broiler, melt the chocolate and butter or coconut oil, mixing together until smooth.

3. Remove from heat and, using a spatula, pour into a medium mixing bowl.

4. Stir in the monk-fruit powder or Swerve, salt, ginger, and almond extract.

5. Allow the mixture to cool slightly.

6. In a new bowl, lightly whisk the eggs, then add the almond flour and tapioca starch.

7. Add the chocolate mixture, and whisk to combine.

8. If using, add toasted walnuts or toasted slivered almonds, and fold into batter.

9. Pour batter into the prepared baking pan. Bake for 30 minutes or until inserted toothpick comes out clean. Store leftovers in an airtight container at room temperature for 3 to 4 days.

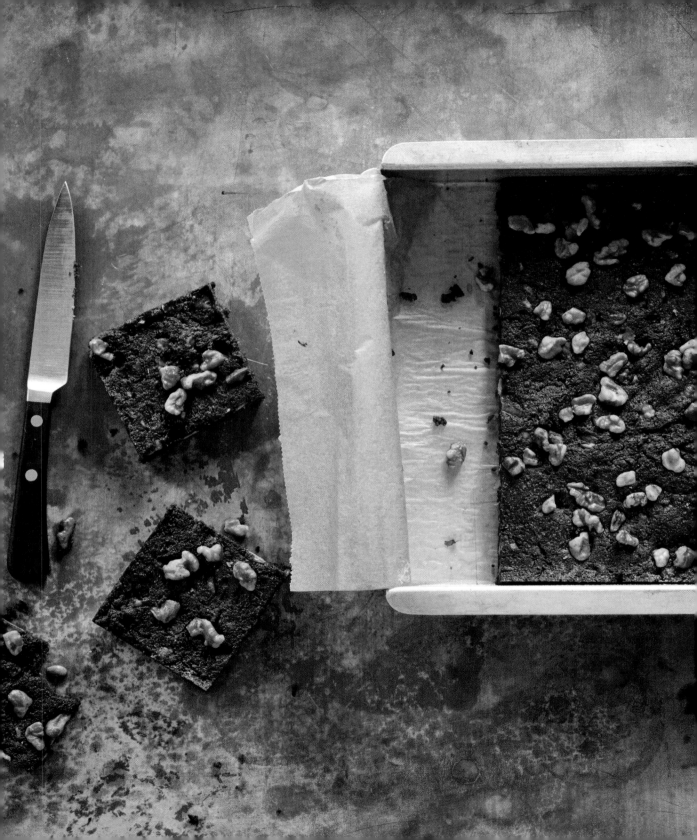

Cinnamon Sweet Potato Blondies

I created this recipe in the fall, when I was feeling a little left out of pumpkin-spice mania. Think of it as a cross between a pumpkin muffin and a blondie—very moist, slightly crisp on top, with warming spices of cinnamon and cloves. Try topping with a dollop of coconut cream for over-the-top deliciousness!

MAKES 12

olive or coconut oil spray

⅓ cup coconut oil, softened but not melted

⅓ cup yacón syrup or 4 tablespoons confectioner's Swerve (erythritol)

½ cup sweet potato puree (from baked sweet potatoes)

1 cup coconut milk

2 omega-3 or pastured eggs or VeganEggs

2 cups blanched almond flour

3 tablespoon coconut flour

½ teaspoon baking soda

1 teaspoon cinnamon

¼ teaspoon cloves

½ teaspoon vanilla extract

½ teaspoon salt

1. Preheat the oven to 350°F. Grease an 8 × 8-inch glass baking dish with olive or coconut oil.

2. Using a whisk in a mixing bowl, or in a stand mixer with a paddle attachment, cream together the coconut oil and yacón syrup (or Swerve).

3. Mix in the sweet potato puree, coconut milk, and eggs.

4. Add the flours, baking soda, spices, vanilla extract, and salt and mix well.

5. Spread the batter evenly in the prepared baking dish.

6. Bake for about 45 minutes, or until a toothpick inserted into the center comes out clean, and the tops are golden brown.

7. Let cool to room temperature before cutting. Store at room temperature in an air-tight container for 3 to 4 days.

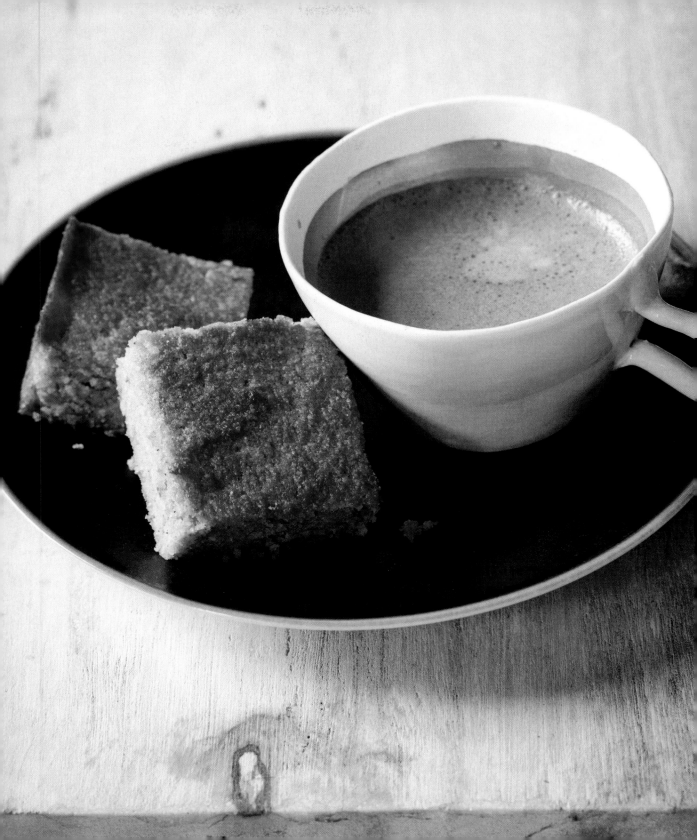

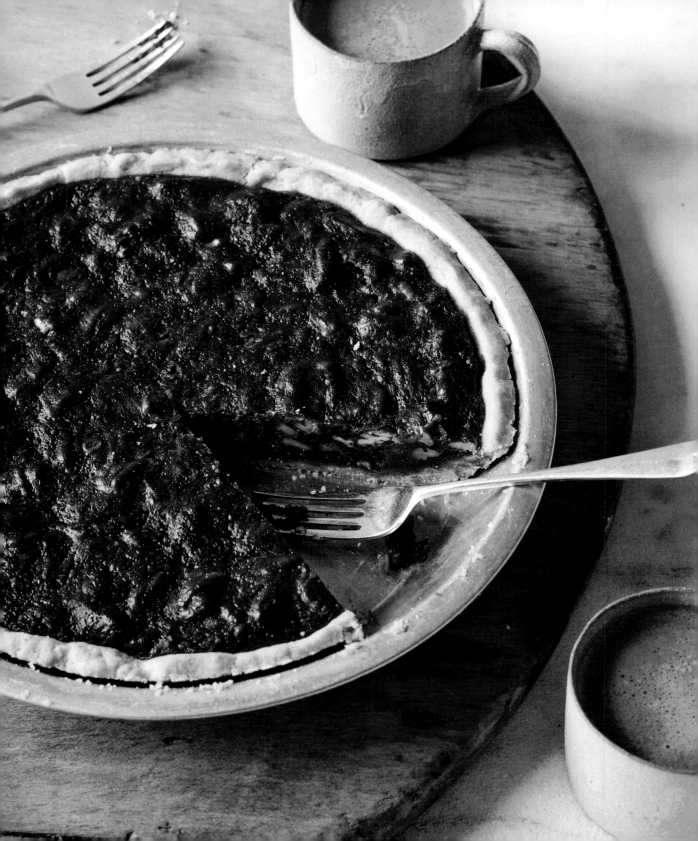

Pecan Pie

Even if you grew up eating your grandmother's version of this Southern staple, I promise my pecan pie will not disappoint. I use monk fruit and dates to give it all of the sweetness of the original, but unlike some traditional versions, this pie isn't cloying. Bourbon and chocolate add layers of flavor that complement the nuts perfectly.

MAKES 1 PIE WITH 8 SERVINGS

1 recipe Plant Paradox Piecrust (page 238), warmed in the oven

5 tablespoons unsalted butter or coconut oil

1 cup monk-fruit sweetener (use a spice grinder to powder) or ½ cup Swerve (erythritol)

½ cup yacón syrup or ¼ cup pureed dates

2¼ ounces bittersweet chocolate (at least 85 percent cacao, if possible), melted

½ teaspoon iodized sea salt

2 cups pecans, toasted and chopped

1½ tablespoons bourbon or vanilla extract

2 teaspoons almond extract

2 omega-3 or pastured eggs or VeganEggs, lightly beaten*

1 egg white*

1 teaspoon tapioca starch

1. Preheat the oven to 350°F.

2. In medium saucepan, combine the butter or coconut oil, monk-fruit sweetener or Swerve, yacón syrup or dates, chocolate, and salt.

3. Over medium heat, bring to a boil, stirring constantly. Continue to stir and boil for about 1 minute.

4. Remove from heat, and add the toasted nuts, bourbon or vanilla extract, and almond extract. Set this mixture aside to cool slightly, about 5 minutes.

5. Once mixture is cooled, whisk in the beaten eggs, egg white (if using), and tapioca starch until you've made a smooth batter.

6. Pour the mixture into the warmed piecrust.

7. Bake on the lower oven rack for 30 minutes, then check to see if the edges of the crust are getting too browned. If they are, cover the entire pie with foil. If they aren't, skip the foil.

8. Bake for an additional 10 to 15 minutes, until the edges of the pie filling are slightly set but the center is still soft or loose, and the edges of the piecrust are lightly brown.

9. Cool pie only slightly once done; it's best served when still warm. Store leftovers in an airtight container at room temperature for 3 to 4 days.

Use 3 VeganEggs instead of the eggs and egg whites.

Plant Paradox Piecrust

This piecrust comes together so easily it's as simple as . . . well, you know. I suggest rolling it out a little thicker than you would roll a traditional piecrust, to prevent cracking during the baking process.

MAKES 2 SINGLE CRUSTS OR 1 DOUBLE CRUST

1½ cups plus 1 tablespoon blanched almond flour

1½ cups plus 1 tablespoon tapioca starch

½ teaspoon monk-fruit sweetener (using spice grinder to make into powder) or 1 packet stevia

½ teaspoon baking powder

½ teaspoon iodized sea salt

1 large omega-3 or pastured egg or VeganEgg

5½ tablespoons softened Italian or French butter or coconut oil

1 teaspoon champagne vinegar or white balsamic vinegar

2 tablespoons cold water, or as needed

1. In a food processor, combine the almond flour, tapioca starch, monk-fruit sweetener (or stevia), baking powder, and salt. Pulse to mix, occasionally using a utensil to scrape down sides.

2. In a small mixing bowl, whisk the egg, butter or coconut oil, and vinegar together.

3. Slowly pour into the food processor while running it on low.

4. Combine and pulse approximately 1 minute; the dough will still look crumbly.

5. Open the food processor and squeeze the dough with your hands to make sure it holds its shape. If it is too dry, add cold water, one teaspoon at a time, and continue to test the dough.

6. Remove the dough from the processor and lightly knead into a ball.

7. If it is too wet and sticky, add some tapioca starch and knead into it.

8. Divide the dough into two equal portions.*

1. Preheat the oven to 350°F. Spray a pie pan liberally with olive oil, and set aside.

2. Between 2 sheets of parchment paper, use a rolling pin to roll out the dough into an even circle to match the size or your pan.

3. Remove top parchment paper and place pie pan on top. Carefully slide your hand under the bottom parchment paper and put your other hand on the pie pan, then flip the dough over while placing it within the pie pan.

4. With the parchment paper still on the dough, mold the dough to the pie pan.

5. Mend any cracks with your finger, then pierce the inside edge where wall of pan starts with a fork. Also pierce 4 times on the bottom (to prevent bubbling).

6. Preheat the oven to 350°F and bake for approximately 30 to 40 minutes, or until lightly brown.

* Dough can be stored, tightly wrapped, for up to 3 days in the fridge or 3 months in the freezer. Allow to thaw overnight before using, if frozen.

chapter twelve

Drinks

BASIL-MINT SPARKLING LEMONADE

CITRUS "SODA"

POMEGRANATE LIME SPRITZER

DR. G'S PLANT-POWERED COFFEE

COCONUT MOCHA

MOCHA "MILKSHAKE"

HAZELNUT VANILLA MILK

Basil-Mint Sparkling Lemonade

Basil is one of my favorite herbs for its health benefits as much as its versatile flavor—it really is one of the rare herbs that enhances both sweet and savory dishes. It also pairs perfectly with citrus, as you'll discover in this refreshing drink. It's also delicious made with fresh lime juice!

SERVES 1

2 to 3 basil leaves

2 to 3 mint leaves

1 slice of lemon

Juice of 1 lemon

5 to 6 drops vanilla stevia

1½ cups sparkling mineral water

1. In the bottom of a large glass, muddle the basil, the mint, and the lemon slice until very fragrant and aromatic.

2. Juice the lemon into the glass and whisk in stevia with a fork.

3. Top with the sparkling water.

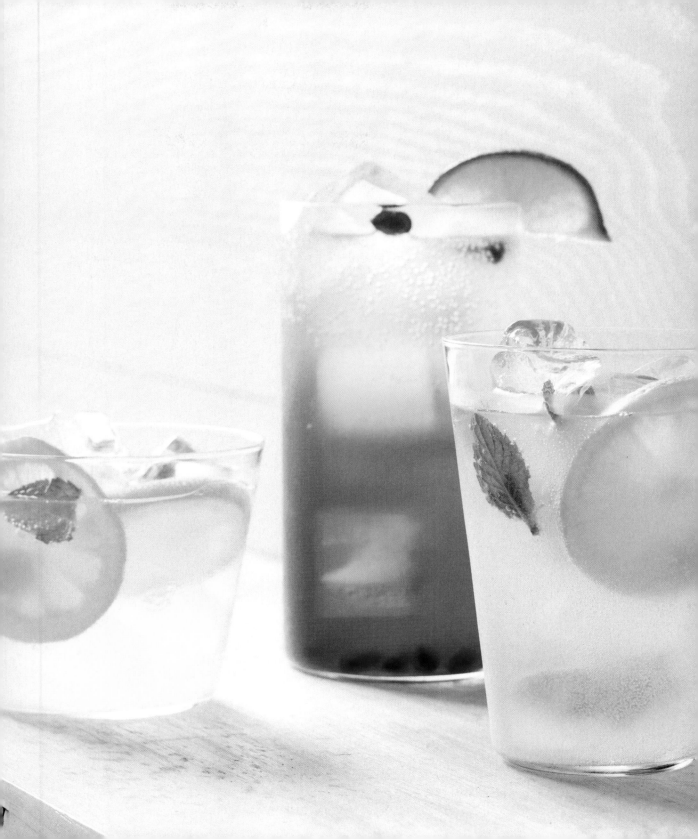

Citrus "Soda"

There is nothing like this sparkling citrus drink to perk up your energy and your mood on a warm day. The orange zest adds a sweetness and delicious orange aroma that is worth the extra effort—don't skip it!

SERVES 1

Juice of ½ lemon

Juice of 1 lime

Zest of ½ orange

4 to 5 mint leaves

4 to 5 drops stevia

2 cups sparkling mineral water

1. Combine the lemon juice, lime juice, orange zest, mint leaves, and stevia in the bottom of a large glass. Stir with a fork.

2. Add the quarter cup of sparkling water and stir.

3. Add ice, if desired, then top off with the rest of the sparkling water.

Pomegranate-Lime Spritzer

If you've never tried pomegranate molasses, I suggest getting a bottle immediately. It's super-concentrated pomegranate juice, and a tiny bit goes a long way. If your grocery store doesn't carry it, try your local Middle Eastern market, or order it online. One bottle will last you a long time!

SERVES 1

Juice of ½ lime

1½ teaspoons pomegranate molasses

2 cups sparkling mineral water

1. Combine the lime juice and the pomegranate molasses in a large glass.

2. Top with sparkling water and give it a stir. Add ice, if desired.

Dr. G's Plant-Powered Coffee

A recent study found that olive oil amplifies the benefits of the polyphenols found in chocolate, so I wanted to make sure to include an olive-oil-and-chocolate recipe in this book. This nutrient-packed coffee drink is the perfect way to start your day. Not a coffee fan? Try it with water, or double the coconut milk.

SERVES 1

2 tablespoons non-Dutched cocoa powder, or 1 scoop GundryMD Heart Defense

1 packet powdered stevia

1 cup unsweetened coconut milk

2 tablespoons extra-virgin olive oil

1 cup cold brew coffee, or water

½ cup ice cubes

1. Place the cocoa powder (or Heart Defense), stevia, and coconut milk in a high-speed blender, and combine with a quick pulse or two, 3 to 5 seconds total.

2. Add the olive oil and coffee, and blend to combine.

3. Add the ice cubes and pulse until cubes are crushed (like one of those fancy frozen coffee house drinks).

4. Serve immediately.

Coconut Mocha

It can be hard to resist the siren song of those sweetened drinks from your neighborhood coffee shop. The good news is, you can get the flavor you crave at home—and save a few bucks in the process! This drink works well hot or iced, and it's a satisfying way to get your caffeine fix.

SERVES 1

1 cup unsweetened coconut milk

1 tablespoon chopped bittersweet chocolate (80 percent cacao is ideal)

2 to 3 drops vanilla stevia or vanilla extract

1 cup very strong black coffee

FOR A HOT DRINK

1. In a small saucepan, heat the coconut milk until simmering.

2. Remove from heat and whisk in the chocolate until melted.

3. Add the vanilla stevia or extract, then stir in the coffee.

4. Serve hot.

FOR AN ICED DRINK

1. Allow the coffee to cool to room temperature.

2. Melt the chocolate in a microwave or over a double boiler.

3. In a high-speed blender, combine all the ingredients, plus 5 or 6 ice cubes.

4. Serve immediately.

Mocha "Milkshake"

This frothy treat is a great way to use up leftover coffee. Once it's cooled to room temperature, just pour into an ice cube tray and freeze to make coffee ice cubes. Not a coffee fan? Freeze 1 cup of coconut milk in an ice cube tray and make a classic chocolate milkshake instead.

SERVES 1

1 cup coffee ice cubes (freeze leftover coffee in a tray)

½ frozen green banana

1 cup unsweetened coconut milk

½ avocado

2 tablespoons cocoa powder

5 to 6 drops vanilla stevia

1. Combine all the ingredients in a high-speed blender and pulse until smooth.

2. Taste, and add stevia as needed.

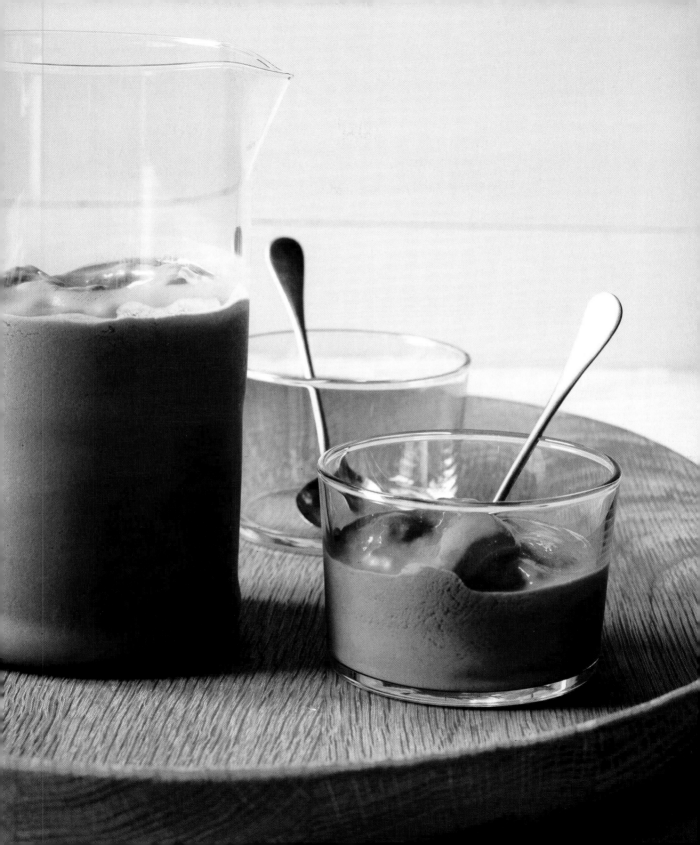

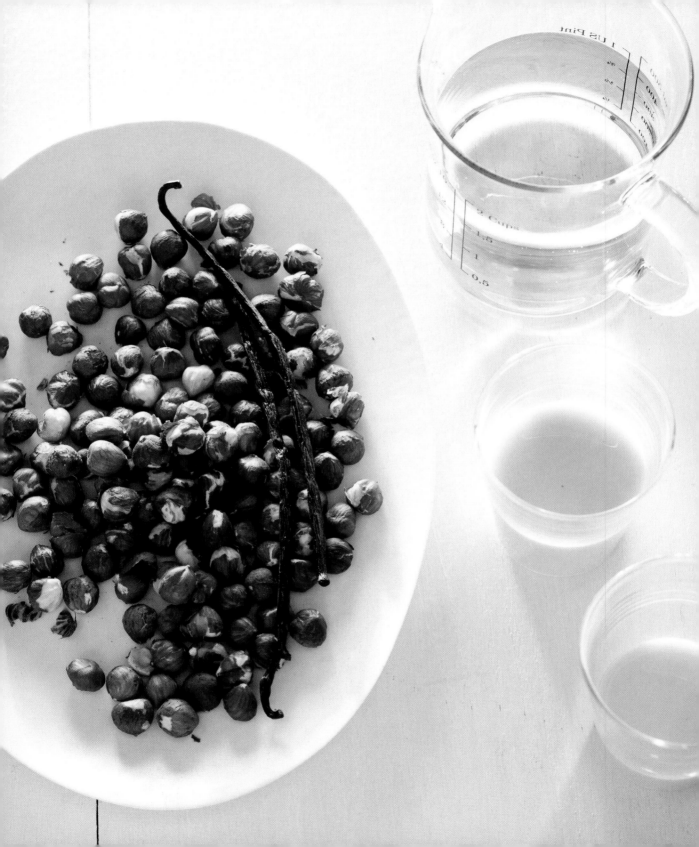

Hazelnut Vanilla Milk

If you're avoiding cow's milk, it's nice to have a flavorful alternative—but so many of the nut milks on the market are high in sugar and contain chemical additives. That's why I love making hazelnut milk at home. To make it really special, I add a little vanilla for sweetness. Bonus: You'll be left with hazelnut meal, which is great for baking.

SERVES 3

2 cups roasted hazelnuts*

1 vanilla bean, split

¼ teaspoon iodized sea salt

3½ cups filtered water, plus 2 cups for soaking overnight

1. Soak the nuts, vanilla bean, and salt in 2 cups of water overnight.

2. Drain and rinse, then transfer to a high-speed blender, like a Vitamix or a Blendtec.

3. Blend for about 2 minutes.

4. Line a fine mesh strainer with a cheesecloth, and strain the blended nuts into a pitcher.

5. Gather the edges of the cheesecloth and squeeze out any excess liquid. Set aside hazelnut meal.

6. Repeat steps 4 and 5 until you've strained out all the liquid from all the milk.

7. Let the hazelnut meal dry, then store in a glass jar in the freezer (and use later in baking, if you'd like). Store milk in the refrigerator for up to a week.

You can make this recipe with any Plant Paradox–approved nut, such as roasted pistachios or pecans, but hazelnuts and vanilla are completely made for one another—and they go great in coffee.

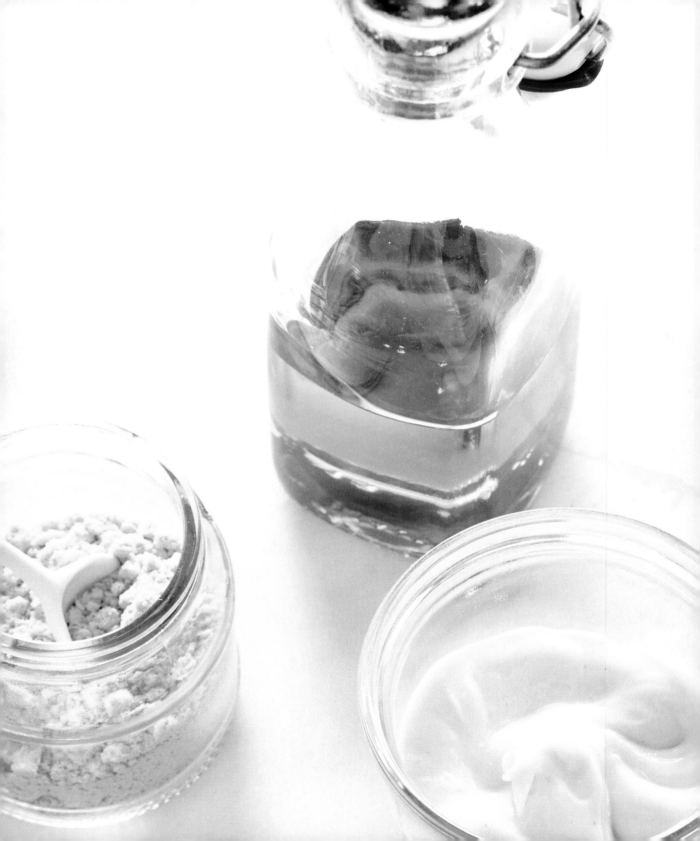

chapter thirteen

Sauces, Condiments, and Dressings

Addictive Caramelized Onion Bourbon Jam

Sometimes I skip traditional dinner and make a cheese plate instead, serving it with a little jam to make it feel more special. I used to go for sour cherry or sugary fig jam, but this caramelized onion jam is even better, and doesn't contain any added sugar.

MAKES 3 CUPS

½ cup sliced nitrate-free pastured bacon (optional)

¼ cup extra-virgin olive oil

6 large yellow onions, thinly sliced

¼ cup fresh thyme leaves

1 teaspoon iodized sea salt

3 tablespoons bourbon or balsamic vinegar

1 tablespoon yacón syrup, or 2 packets stevia

1. If using bacon, sauté it over medium-low heat until slightly crispy. Add the oil, onions, thyme, and salt to a skillet over medium-low heat. Stir regularly to prevent burning.

2. Cook for 20 to 30 minutes, until onions are richly golden brown.

3. Add the bourbon or vinegar and sweetener and cook until all liquid disappears.

4. Transfer to the mixture to jars and let cool before serving. Jam will keep 2 to 3 weeks in the refrigerator.

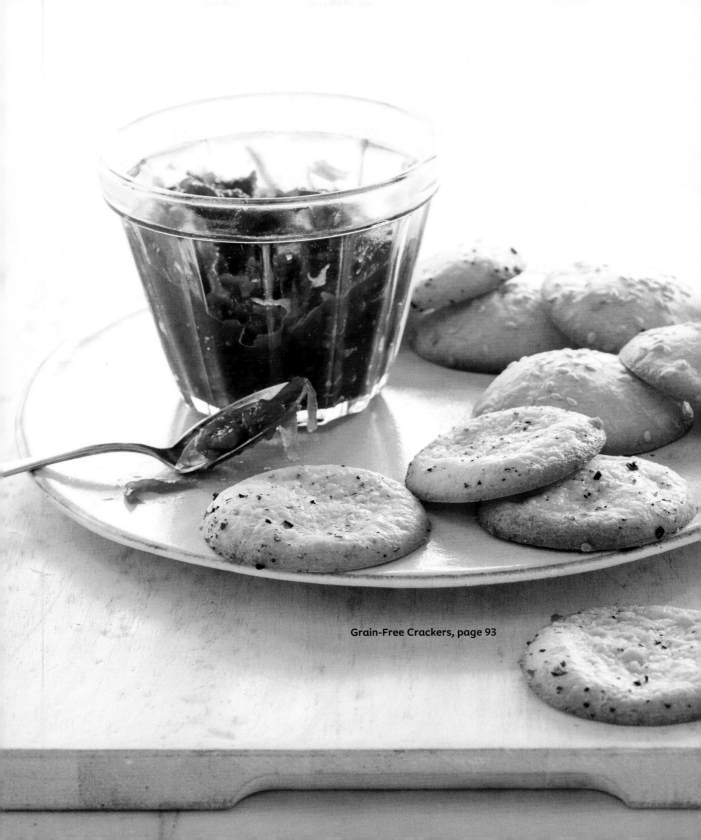

Grain-Free Crackers, page 93

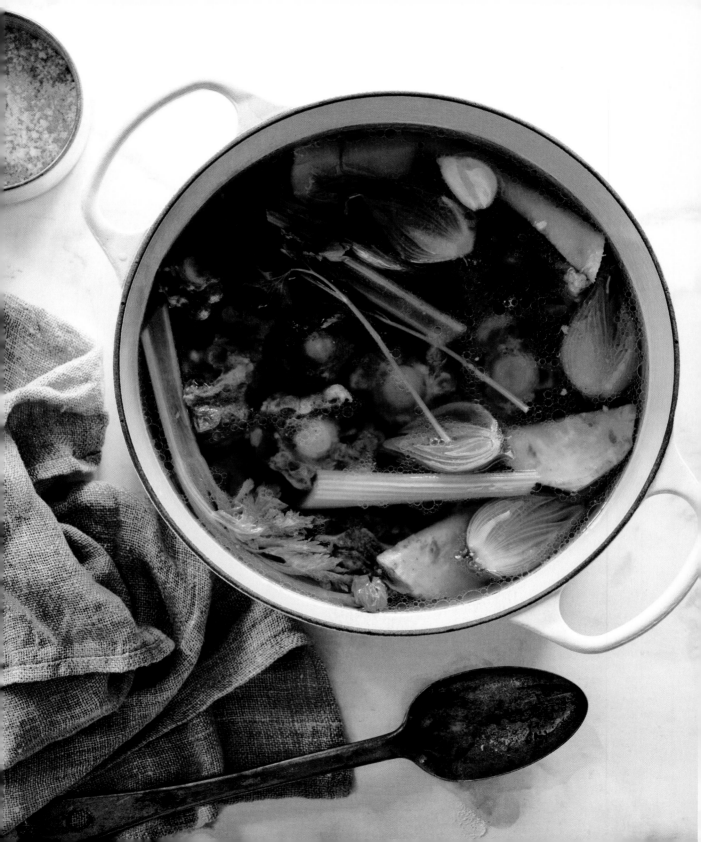

Bone Broth

Most commercially available bone broth is made from livestock that's fed a diet of lectin- and GMO-heavy grains. Luckily, it's easy to make your own at home. When you do, you can be sure to use the bones of pastured animals.

NUMBER OF SERVINGS VARIES

4 pounds bones and gelatinous parts of animals (cartilage, etc.)*

1 medium celery root, roughly chopped

1 parsnip, roughly chopped

2 medium celery stalks

1 cup aromatics (see chart below)

1 medium white onion, skin on

5 cloves garlic, peeled

2 tablespoon apple cider vinegar or fresh lemon juice

2 to 3 bay leaves

1 tablespoon iodized sea salt

Enough water to cover the bones, but no more than ⅔ capacity of your pressure cooker or ¾ capacity of your stockpot or slow cooker

1. Add all the ingredients to a pressure cooker, slow cooker, or stockpot.

2. If pressure-cooking: Cook for 90 minutes, according to manufacturer's instructions. Release pressure.

   If slow-cooking: Cook for 10 hours on low.

   If cooking on stove: Cook for 6 to 8 hours on medium-low heat, covered.

3. Pour broth through a strainer to remove bones and vegetables. Strain a second time (through a fine mesh strainer), then use immediately or refrigerate.**

* For a vegetarian broth, use mushrooms instead—either 2 cups dried or 4 cups fresh, or 3 cups total if using a mixture of both.

** This broth should gel in the refrigerator—that's a sign you extracted lots of collagen from the bones. Don't be alarmed!

MEAT	AROMATICS
Pastured chicken—feet, legs, skin, neck	Fennel, parsley, shallots, lemon zest
Pastured or acorn-fed pork—feet, ribs	Orange, cinnamon sticks, thyme, apple
Pastured beef—oxtail, short ribs	Red wine, parsley, rosemary, shallots
Kosher turkey—necks, feet, wings	Sage, apple, shallots, thyme

Classic Basil Pesto

There are a million pesto recipes out there, but this is my hands-down favorite. I encourage using pine nuts whenever possible, but if they're not available (or affordable), blanched almonds work well as a substitute. Just make sure to toast them well!

MAKES 1 CUP

½ cup toasted pine nuts or blanched toasted almonds

3 cloves garlic

1 teaspoon iodized sea salt

½ cup grated Parmigiano-Reggiano cheese or ¼ cup nutritional yeast

3 cups fresh basil leaves, loosely packed

¾ cup top quality extra-virgin olive oil

1. In a high-speed blender or a food processor fitted with an S-blade, pulse together the nuts, garlic, and sea salt until powdery.

2. Add cheese and basil and pulse to combine, scraping occasionally.

3. With motor running, drizzle in olive oil until fully incorporated.

4. Use immediately, or store in an airtight container for up to a week in the refrigerator.

5. If you want to store your pesto longer, transfer it into ice cube trays and pop it in the freezer. Once frozen, transfer the cubes to an air-tight freezer bag.

* For a fun twist, try pistachios instead of the almonds or pine nuts, and add lemon zest. You can also substitute some of the basil with mint or parsley.

Plant Paradox Guacamole

I love guacamole, but here's a secret about me: I'm one of those people who doesn't enjoy the flavor of cilantro (it's actually not a matter of taste . . . it's a genetic predisposition). I recognize that I'm in the minority, so this version includes it. But if you're cilantro-averse like me, try substituting with flat-leaf parsley and mint leaves instead.

SERVES 4 TO 6

4 ripe avocados, cut in half, pits removed

2 cloves garlic, crushed

1 red onion, minced

¼ cup cilantro

1 teaspoon cumin

1 teaspoon iodized sea salt

Juice of 4 limes

1 dash of hot sauce (optional)

1. Spoon the avocado into a large bowl, and mash with a potato masher (even on the Plant Paradox plan, they come in handy).

2. Add the remaining ingredients to the bowl and stir well to combine.

3. Taste and adjust seasoning as needed.

4. Serve with your choice of sliced jicama, raw carrots, Cassava Tortillas (and Chips) (page 36), or Siete brand grain-free tortilla chips.

Fool Proof Salad Dressing

Once you know a good basic vinaigrette, it's easy to make any salad taste great. Mine is more of a formula than a recipe, which makes it incredibly versatile. This dressing is a touch more acidic than the standard vinaigrette, but if you like it milder, increase the oil to three-quarters of a cup.

MAKES 1 CUP

½ cup oil (such as extra-virgin olive oil or avocado oil)

½ cup acid (such as balsamic vinegar, champagne vinegar, or red wine vinegar)

1½ teaspoon Dijon mustard

Seasonings, as needed

1. Add all ingredients to a high-speed blender and blend until emuslified, or whisk it together by hand.

2. Use right away or store in a jar with a tight-fitting lid, so you can shake it up before serving.

Really, the possibilities are endless, and that's half the fun. Try adding your favorite herbs, mixing in your favorite oil (or yogurt), or switching up the vinegar for citrus juice. You may discover a new favorite!

CLASSIC BALSAMIC VINAIGRETTE

½ cup extra-virgin olive oil

¼ cup balsamic vinegar

¼ cup lemon juice

1½ teaspoons mustard

1 clove crushed garlic

1 teaspoon minced fresh rosemary

OR, FOR A CREAMIER DRESSING

½ avocado

¼ cup lemon juice

¼ cup white balsamic vinegar

1½ teaspoons mustard

2 tablespoons fresh parsley

1 clove crushed garlic

ASIAN-INSPIRED DRESSING

½ cup toasted sesame oil

¼ cup lime juice

¼ cup rice wine vinegar

1½ teaspoons mustard

1 crushed clove garlic

1 teaspoon grated fresh ginger

1 dash coconut aminos

GOT LEFTOVER PESTO?

¼ cup extra-virgin olive oil

¼ cup basil pesto

¼ cup white balsamic vinegar

¼ cup lemon juice

1½ teaspoons mustard

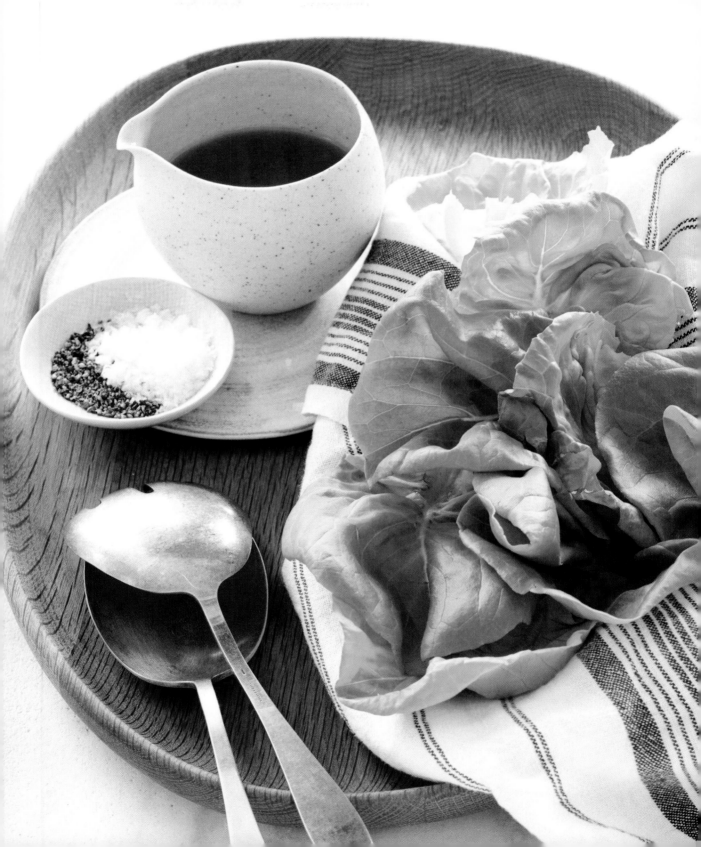

Mayonnaise, Two Ways

Classic mayo isn't inherently bad for you as long as you make it with the right ingredients. But if you're not a mayo person, or if you avoid eggs, I've also included a vegan avocado mayo recipe here. You can technically leave out the garlic in both of these recipes for a more traditional flavor—but why?

MAKES 1 CUP

CLASSIC MAYONNAISE

3 large egg yolks from omega-3 or pasture-raised eggs

1 clove garlic

¼ teaspoon Dijon mustard

1 teaspoon dry mustard

¼ teaspoon salt

1 tablespoon lemon juice

¾ cup extra-virgin olive oil

VEGAN MAYONNAISE

1 medium to large avocado

Juice of ½ lemon

1 clove garlic, crushed

¼ teaspoon salt

½ teaspoon powdered mustard

½ cup extra-virgin olive oil

CLASSIC MAYONNAISE

1. Place the eggs, garlic, mustard and mustard powder, salt, and lemon juice into the carafe of a high-speed blender.

2. Gradually increase speed to high until the garlic is broken into tiny pieces and the mixture is well-combined.

3. Reduce speed to medium. While blender is running, drizzle the oil into the mixture.

4. Continue to blend for about 30 seconds, until mixture start to thicken.

5. Refrigerate and use within 2 to 4 weeks.

VEGAN MAYONNAISE

1. Add the avocado, lemon juice, garlic, salt, and mustard powder to a high-speed blender and blend until smooth.

2. With blender running, stream in the olive oil until mixture is well-combined.

3. Serve immediately, or refrigerate for 3 to 4 days.

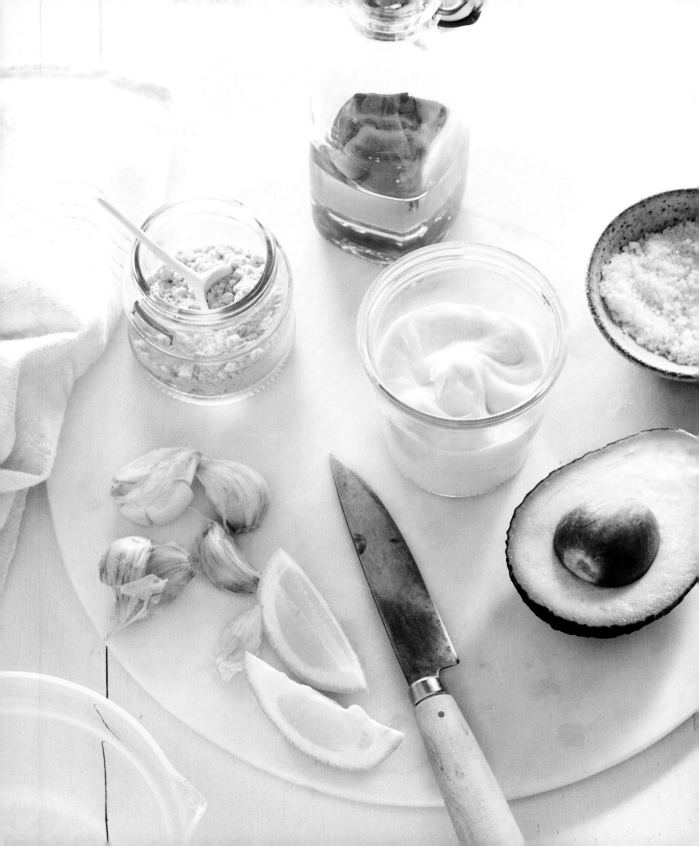

Vegan Caesar Dressing

This recipe is an update on my Seed-Sar Salad from *Dr. Gundry's Diet Evolution*. It's a vegan twist on a classic Caesar dressing, and while it's delicious on salad, it's a versatile addition to many dishes: try it tossed with cauliflower rice, in a lettuce wrap or on a sandwich, or even tossed with sautéed greens and Miracle noodles.

MAKES 1 CUP

½ cup tahini

1 garlic clove, crushed

¼ teaspoon iodized sea salt

¼ teaspoon crushed black pepper

Juice of 1 lemon

1 teaspoon Dijon mustard

¼ cup extra-virgin olive oil

1 dash coconut aminos

1. Whisk together all the ingredients in a bowl until smooth and well-combined.

2. Serve immediately, or refrigerate up to 1 week.

Vegetable Stock

Once you know how to make a flavorful, well-balanced vegetable stock, it'll be hard to go back to the store-bought stuff. You can really use any vegetables you've got on hand, but don't skip the onions—they're the key to building flavor.

NUMBER OF SERVINGS VARIES

¼ cup extra-virgin olive oil

2 onions, diced

2 parsnips, diced

4 celery stalks, diced

1 bulb fennel, chopped

1 cup mushrooms, chopped

4 cloves garlic, crushed

4 to 5 sprigs fresh thyme

1 bay leaf

1 small bunch parsley

1 teaspoon whole peppercorns

Juice of 1 lemon

1 tablespoon iodized sea salt

Enough water to cover vegetables

1. In a large stockpot, heat the olive oil over medium-high heat.

2. Add the onions, parsnips, celery, fennel, and mushrooms, and sauté until the onions begin to become translucent and fragrant.

3. Add the remaining ingredients. Cover the pot, and simmer on low for 30 to 45 minutes.

4. Strain twice, then use immediately or freeze for up to 6 months.

Lectin-Fighting Shellfish Broth

The shells of shrimp, crawfish, and other shellfish have lectin-blocking powers, and one of the best ways to harness them is through a simple shellfish broth like this one. Tip: When you're using shrimp in a recipe, save the shells in a container in your freezer. When you have enough, make this broth!

SERVES 4 TO 6

1 tablespoon extra-virgin olive oil

4 cups shrimp shells (from 2 pounds shrimp, fresh or frozen)

1 unpeeled red onion, sliced

2 celery stalks, sliced

1 bulb shallot, sliced

3 garlic cloves, smashed

1 sprig parsley

1 sprig thyme

1 sprig tarragon

1 to 2 bay leaves

1 teaspoon saffron (optional, but lovely)

1 teaspoon iodized sea salt

6 cups water, or enough to cover

1. In a stockpot, heat the olive oil over medium heat. Add the shells and cook for 10 minutes.

2. Add all the remaining ingredients except the water.

3. Turn heat to medium-high, and cook, uncovered, for about 10 minutes.

4. Cover and cook for an additional 10 minutes.

5. Add the water to the pot and bring to a boil, then simmer for 20 minutes.

6. Strain into a heat-proof container.

7. Use immediately, or let cool to room temperature before freezing for up to 6 months.

Resources

For More Information Online

GUNDRYMD.COM

This is my personal website, where I post my thoughts, videos, breaking health news, and recipes to keep you motivated and inspired. It's also where I sell the supplements I have painstakingly developed to help support the health of myself, my family, and my patients.

DR. GUNDRY FACEBOOK PAGE (https://www.facebook.com/GundryMD/)

Follow me on Facebook to not only get recipes and articles delivered to your news feed but also to meet other folks like you who are devoted to eating the Plant Paradox way.

Supplements

It's my firm belief that even if you have the most immaculate, health-promoting diet, you can still benefit from the right supplements. Why? Because modern farming practices, such as the use of pesticides, herbicides, and chemical fertilizers, have depleted our soil of nutrients and friendly bacterial populations. You simply can't get all the nutrients and micronutrients you need from food, because the food you eat isn't able to deliver those nutrients from the soil.

In my own life and in my practice with the thousands of patients I have seen, these are the supplements I recommend, because these vitamins and minerals are essential to our well-being, and the vast majority of us are deficient in them:

VITAMIN D

Even here in sunny Southern California, about 80 percent of my patients are vitamin D deficient when I first begin treating them, and that number is closer to 100 percent if those patients have an autoimmune disorder. This is a serious problem, because vitamin D plays an important role in helping your immune system to function, your bones to stay strong, and your beneficial intestinal flora and gut wall to be healthy. I recommend that everyone take at least 5,000 IUs of vitamin D3 daily, and if you have an autoimmune condition, make that 10,000.

B VITAMINS

B vitamins are key for protecting the inner lining of your blood vessels, and about half the population has a genetic mutation that prevents them from being able to convert folic acid and vitamin B12 into their active forms. To make sure you are getting enough B vitamins in a form that your body can use, I recommend taking methylfolate (the active form of folic acid), 1,000 mcg a day, and methyl B12 (the active form of vitamin B12), 1,000 to 5,000 mcg under your tongue each day.

GREEN PLANT PHYTOCHEMICALS

Your gut buddies love greens, but you have to take care not to take a greens supplement that contains lectin-rich grasses such as wheatgrass, barley grass, or oat grass. The supplements I recommend to lend you the vibrance of eating large amount of greens are:

- Spinach extract, 1,000 mg

- DIM (diindolylmethane), an immune-boosting compound found in broccoli, 100 mg

- Primal Plants, a supplement available on GundryMD.com, that combines spinach extract, DIM, and ten other superfood greens

POLYPHENOLS

These phytochemicals protect plants from insects and sun damage, and they offer many benefits to you, including improved cardiovascular health and support of your gut bacteria. The polyphenol-containing supplements I recommend taking daily (you can choose one, or take a combination) are:

- Grape seed extract, 100 mg

- Pine tree bark extract, 25 to 100 mg

- Resveratrol (the polyphenol in red wine)

- Or you can take Vital Reds, my own blend of polyphenols that I sell at

GundryMD.com, which contains thirty-four polyphenols total, including green tea extract, berberine, cinnamon, mulberry, and pomegranate, as well as my favorite probiotic.

PREBIOTICS

Prebiotics are the substances that feed and nourish your gut buddies—they are the fertilizer that boosts the health of your internal garden. In addition to supporting your immunity, prebiotics will help to keep you regular. Good prebiotic supplements include:

- Psyllium husks, a teaspoon a day in water, working up to a tablespoon per day

- Inulin powder, a teaspoon a day (the sweetener Just Like Sugar is primarily inulin)

- PrebioThrive, a combination of five prebiotics that I formulated and sell on GundryMD.com. It's a powder that you mix with water and drink every day.

LECTIN BLOCKERS

Remember, you can't avoid all lectins in your diet. For the lectins you do consume, it helps to have some lectin-fighting compounds in your system. These include:

- Glucosamine, which occurs naturally in the fluid that surrounds and protects your joints and serves a building block of cartilage, binds to inflammatory lectins and reduces pain. You can take one Osteo Bi-Flex or Move Free (both can be found at Costco) daily.

- D-mannose, the active ingredient in cranberries, is also an effective lectin blocker. Take 1,000 mg a day (divided into two doses of 500 mg each).

- Lectin Shield, which is my formulation available on my website, contains nine ingredients that have been proven to block or absorb lectins so that they don't reach your gut wall; you can take two of these before a meal that you suspect will be high in lectins.

SUGAR BLOCKERS

To maintain healthy blood glucose levels, I recommend the following:

- CinSulin, a combination of chromium and cinnamon available at Costco, two capsules a day

- Zinc, 30 mg

- Selenium, 150 mcg

- Berberine, 250 mg twice a day

- Turmeric extract, 200 mg twice a day

- Glucose Defense, a product I formulated and sell at GundryMD.com, covers all these bases by combining chromium, zinc, selenium, cinnamon bark extract, berberine, turmeric extract, and black pepper extract (for better absorbability), two capsules twice a day.

OMEGA-3S

Omega-3 fats are vital to the health of your gut and the health of your brain. In fact, half the fat in your brain—which is made up of 60 percent fat in total—is a long-chain omega-3 fat called DHA. Yes, in my ten years of seeing patients, nearly everyone is majorly deficient in these vital fats. Unless you're eating sardines or herring on a daily basis, you likely need to take an omega-3 supplement. I recommend:

- Fish oil, molecularly distilled and from small fish such as sardines and anchovies, enough to get 1,000 mg of DHA per day. Brands I like include Kirkland Signature Fish Oil (enteric coated, for no fish burps), OmegaVia DHA 600, and Carlson Elite Omega-3 Gems.

Acknowledgments

The Plant Paradox Cookbook could not have happened without the incredible outpouring of support and recipes and requests from all of you who took the teachings of The Plant Paradox program and wanted it to be a way of life. And wanted more recipes ASAP! And that required assembling a dedicated team who answered the call to produce the beautiful book you have in your hands. It holds my recipes; your recipes, dear readers; recipes from my patients, many of whom have lived this lifestyle for years; and most importantly, the recipes developed at GundryMD by my collaborator and head chef extraordinaire, Kathryn "Kate" Holzhauer. Kate makes me and all my GundryMD YouTube segments look great and makes the food taste great, and now she's taken her talents to a new level! She not only designed and perfected so many of the dishes contained in this book, but also painstakingly tested all the other submissions for ease of use. I think you will find out after just one recipe how easy it is to live a lectin-free lifestyle without giving up the tastes and textures you love. Thank you, Kate!

Speaking of Kate, my thanks go to another Kate, Kate Hanley, who was able to take my very lengthy prose and writing style and condense it into an easy and quick to understand summary of my principles in *The Plant Paradox* for this cookbook. Even if you never got around to reading that book (I hope you will!), you have all the tools and knowledge you need to get started cooking today.

My deep thanks go to my longtime friends and fellow dreamers, the great James Beard Award–winning chefs Jimmy Schmidt and Jonathan Waxman, the latter of Jams and Barbuto fame, both of whom had their lives impacted by limiting lectins, and who were kind enough to lend some of their most popular recipes, reworked, to this cookbook. And thank you to celebrated chef and dear friend, Tara Lazar, from the Palm Springs hip dining scene, where scores of people wait patiently for hours for a table at Cheeky's or Birba, who contributed the pizza that graces the cover and will soon grace your tummy! To Ralph Skidmore and Steve Pargman and Pamela Trevett, Penny's and my good friends, who daily live the Plant Paradox lifestyle, your recipes and friendship are so appreciated! Thanks again to my friend and chef Irina Skoeries, who contributed the 3-day Kickstart in *The Plant Paradox* and who now delivers Plant Paradox–compatible meals overnight via CatalystCruisine.com. And to Jessica Murnane, the great vegan authoress who, unlike the naysayers, tried the vegan version of The Plant Paradox and was won over; thanks for your delicious recipe as well. Finally, for the GundryMD recipe contest winners and all you amazing followers who submitted recipes: I'm sorry I couldn't include them all, but, hey, there's always PPC#2, right?

Speaking of recipes, food not only has to taste good but also look good! My great thanks to my photographer Dana Gallaghe, and my food stylist Heather Meldrom, both of whom captured how great food for you and your gut buddies can capture your heart and mind with a picture! And making all this happen, quickly and beautifully, was my project manager from Stonesong, Ellen Scordato. Thank you all, again.

The team at HarperWave did it again without so much as a hiccup in getting this project completed in record time. Thanks again to my now longtime publisher Karen Rinaldi, and Brian Perrin, director of marketing, and Yelena Nesbit, my new publicist. And of course, thanks to my dear editor extraordinaire, Julie Will, who lovingly beat me and *The Plant Paradox* into the major bestseller that has changed so many lives for the better, which, of course, fostered this book.

All this was guided by my longtime agent and early believer, Shannon Marven, president of Dupree Miller, and my attorney and longtime friend and supporter, Dave Baron and his associate Ini Ghidirmic, and my accountant Joyce Ohmura, who were able to corral all these disparate entities into a beautiful finished product.

Like I said in *The Plant Paradox*, I cannot thank individually the entire 500-plus people at GundryMD who have made me and GundryMD.com the trusted source for health and supplement advice for millions of people daily, but I have to single out Lanee Lee Neil, who for the past year has daily, weekends as well, lorded over me and my brand. I couldn't have done it without you! Likewise, Jody Sowa and her team of publicists, including Rebecca Reinbold, and Jessica Hofmann at Stanton Company keep me and GundryMD in the spotlight daily. Thank you, all.

And speaking of couldn't have done it without you, heartfelt thanks to my entire staff at The International Heart and Lung Institute and The Centers for Restorative Medicine in Palm Springs and Santa Barbara, CA! As if things weren't busy enough before "The Plant Paradox," wow, did you guys step up to the plate! Directed by Susan Lokken, my loyal team of Adda Harris, Tanya Marta, Cindy Harpster (who singlehandedly keeps the office afloat monetarily), Donna Fitzgerald, my daughter, Melissa Perko, and of course the "Blood Suckers" led by Laurie Acuna and Lynn Visk, and my new Physician's Assistant, Mitzu Killion-Jacobo. How you keep the chaos controlled is a true testament to your loyalty to the cause of making our patients well.

Speaking of controlling chaos, my real rock in all of this is my wife Penny, who, along with our four dogs, never let me forget that, when the sun rises each day, I'm really only a dog walker and if I do that job well, the rest of the day will follow suit!

Finally, like I said in *The Plant Paradox*, none of this would be possible without you, my patients. Thank you for your trust in me and my team as we together try to maximize our collective knowledge and health.

Endnotes

1   Hermanussen M. Stature of early Europeans. *Hormones*. Jul–Sep, 2003; 2(3): 175–178.

2   Ibid.

3   Abdel-Rahman AA, et al. Splenda alters gut microflora and increases intestinal p-glycoprotein and cytochrome p-450 in male rats. *Journal of Toxicology and Environmental Health*. 2008; 71(21): 1415–1429.

4   International Agency for Research on Cancer, World Health Organization. IARC Monographs, Volume 112: evaluation of five organophosphate insecticides and herbicides. March 20, 2015. https:www.iarc.fr/en/media-centre/iarcnews/pdf/MonographVolume112.pdf, accessed on November 1, 2017.

5   Food Safety: Frequently Asked Questions, *JMPR Secretariat*, May 27, 2016, http://www.who.int/foodsafety/faq/en, accessed on November 21, 2017.

6   Andreotti G, Koutros S, Hofmann JN, et al. Glyphosate use and cancer incidence in the Agricultural Health Study. *Journal of the National Cancer Institute*. 2017.

7   Mesnage R, Renney G, Séralini GE, et al. Multiomics reveal non-alcoholic fatty liver disease in rats following chronic exposure to an ultra-low dose of Roundup herbicide. *Scientific Reports*. 2017; 7: 39328.

8   Kharrazian D, Herbert M, Vojdani A. Detection of islet cell immune reactivity with low glycemic index foods: is this a concern for type 1 diabetes? *Journal of Diabetes Research*. 2017; 2017: 4124967.

9   Załęski A., Banaszkiewicz A., Walkowiak J. Butyric acid in irritable bowel syndrome. *Przeglad Gastroenterologiczny*. 2013; 8(6): 350–353.

10 Wang L, Bordi PL, Fleming JA, et al. Effect of a moderate fat diet with and without avocados on lipoprotein particle number, size and subclasses in overweight and obese adults: a randomized, controlled trial. *Journal of the American Heart Association*. 2015; 4(1): e001355.

11 de Morais CL, Pinheiro SS, Martino HS, Pinheiro-Sant'Ana HM. Sorghum (*Sorghum bicolor L.*): Nutrients, bioactive compounds, and potential impact on human health. *Critical Reviews in Food Science and Nutrition*. 2017; 57(2): 372–390.

12 Saleh ASM, Zhang Q, Chen J, Shen Q. Millet grains: nutritional quality, processing, and potential health benefits. *Comprehensive Reviews in Food Science and Food Safety*. 2013; 12(3): 281–295.

13 Martinez I, Kim J, Duffy PR, et al. Resistant starches types 2 and 4 have differential effects on the composition of the fecal microbiota in human subjects. *PLoS One*. 2010; 5(11): e15046.

14 Wall R, Ross RP, Fitzgerald GF, Stanton C. Fatty acids from fish: the anti-inflammatory potential of long-chain omega-3 fatty acids. *Nutrition Reviews*. 2010; 68(5): 280–289.

15 Ander BP, Dupasquier CMC, Prociuk MA, Pierce GN. Polyunsaturated fatty acids and their effects on cardiovascular disease. *Experimental & Clinical Cardiology*. 2003; 8(4): 164–172.

16 Oh SY, Ryue J, Hsieh CH, Bell DE. Eggs enriched in omega-3 fatty acids and alterations in lipid concentrations in plasma and lipoproteins and in blood pressure. *American Journal of Clinical Nutrition*. 1991; 54(4): 689–695.

17 Samman S, Kung F, Carter L, et al. Fatty acid composition of certified organic, conventional and omega-3 eggs. *Food Chemistry*. 2009; 116(4): 911–914.

18 Pal S, Woodford K, Kukuljan S, Ho S. Milk intolerance, beta-casein and lactose. *Nutrients*. 2015; 7(9): 7285–7297.

19 Kwok CS, Boekholdt SM, Lentjes MA, et al. Habitual chocolate consumption and risk of cardiovascular disease among healthy men and women. *Heart*. 2015; 101(16): 1279–1287.

20 Saleem TM, Basha SD. Red wine: A drink to your heart. *Journal of Cardiovascular Disease Research*. 2010; 1(4): 171–176.

21 Corona G, Vauzour D, Hercelin J, et al. Phenolic acid intake, delivered *via* moderate Champagne wine consumption, improves spatial working memory *via* the modulation of hippocampal and cortical protein expression/activation. *Antioxidants & Redox Signaling*. 2013; 19(14): 1676–1689.

22 Slanina P. Solanine (glycoalkaloids) in potatoes: Toxicological evaluation. *Food and Chemical Toxicology*. 1990; 28(11): 759–761.

23 Cuadrado C, Hajos G, Burbano C, et al. Effect of natural fermentation on the lectin of lentils measured by immunological methods. *Food and Agriculture Immunology*. 2002; 14(1): 41–49.

24 Watch Your Garden Grow: Eggplant, University of Illinois Extension, http://extension.illinois.edu/veggies/eggplant.cfm, accessed on October 12, 2017.

25 Ananieva, E. Targeting amino acid metabolism in cancer growth and anti-tumor immune response. *World Journal of Biological Chemistry*. 2015; 6(4): 281–289.

26 The Low Histamine Chef. 2015. Interview: Fasting mimicking diets for mast cell activation & allergies. https://healinghistamine.com/interview-fasting-mimicking-diets-for-mast-cell-activation-allergies, , accessed on November 10, 2016.

27 Fox, M. Cancer cells slurp up fructose, US study finds. 2010. https://www.reuters.com/article/cancer-fructose-idAFN0210830520100802, accessed on November 22, 2017.

28 David LA, Maurice CF, Carmody RN, et al. Diet rapidly and reproducibly alters the human gut microbiome. *Nature*. 2014; 505(7484): 559-563.

29 Zarrinpar A, Chaix A, Yooseph S, Panda S. Diet and feeding pattern affect the diurnal dynamics of the gut microbiome. *Cell Metabolism*. 2014; 20(6): 1006–1017.

30 Wu GD, Chen J, Hoffmann C, et al. Linking long-term dietary patterns with gut microbial enterotypes. *Science*. 2011; 334(6052): 105–108.

Index

Note: Page numbers in *italic* refer to photos.

About the Author

STEVEN R. GUNDRY, MD, is the director of the International Heart and Lung Institute in Palm Springs, California, and the founder and director of the Center for Restorative Medicine in Palm Springs and Santa Barbara. After a distinguished surgical career as a professor and chairman of cardiothoracic surgery at Loma Linda University, Dr. Gundry changed his focus to curing modern diseases via dietary changes. He is the author of *The Plant Paradox* and *Dr. Gundry's Diet Evolution* as well as more than three hundred articles published in peer-reviewed journals on using diet and supplements to eliminate heart disease, diabetes, autoimmune disease, and multiple other diseases. Dr. Gundry lives with his wife, Penny, and their dogs in Palm Springs and Montecito, California.